RECENT TRENDS IN CARDIOVASCULAR RISKS

Edited by **Arun Kumar**

Recent Trends in Cardiovascular Risks
http://dx.doi.org/10.5772/65843
Edited by Arun Kumar

Contributors

Parinya Chamnan, Wichai Aekplakorn, Jingmei Jiang, Alexandra Mastaleru, Elena Cojocaru, Bogdan Tamba, Roxana Cobzaru, Maria Magdalena Leon, Raluca Georgiana Vasile, Carmen Valerica Ripa, Razvan Cosmin Tudor, Francisco Jose Sanchez Muniz, M Pilar Vaquero, Ángel García-Quismondo, Francisco J. Del Cañizo, Russell Kabir, Sayeeda Rahman, Md. Anwarul Azim Majumder, Subir Gupta, Prasad Dalvi, Nkemcho Ojeh, S.M. Yasir Arafat, Mainul Haque, Arun Kumar

Published by InTech
Janeza Trdine 9, 51000 Rijeka, Croatia

Publishing Process Manager Mirena Calmic
Technical Editor SPi Global
Cover InTech Design team

First published July, 2017
Printed in Croatia
Legal deposit, Croatia: National and University Library in Zagreb

Additional hard copies can be obtained from orders@intechopen.com

Recent Trends in Cardiovascular Risks, Edited by Arun Kumar
p. cm.
Print ISBN 978-953-51-3327-8
Online ISBN 978-953-51-3328-5

For EU product safety concerns:
IN TECH d.o.o., Prolaz Marije Krucifikse Kozulić 3, 51000 Rijeka, Croatia,
info@intechopen.com or visit our website at intechopen.com.

Meet the editor

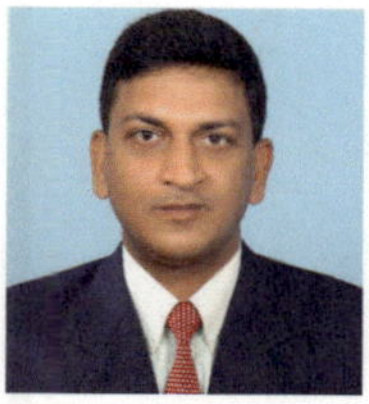

Dr. Arun Kumar has 18 years of teaching experience in Medical Biochemistry at various medical schools in India and abroad. He has published more than 150 scientific articles in national and international indexed journals. He has authored seven books and contribution of chapters in two text books. Currently, he is an editor in chief of several international journals.

His current research interests are dyslipidemia, metabolic syndrome, lipidology, cardiovascular biology, diabetes, and medical education. Dr. Arun Kumar did his graduation and postgraduation from Jawaharlal Institute of Postgraduate Medical Education and Research, Pondicherry, India. He further did his doctorate degree from the University of Peradeniya, Sri Lanka, in Medical Biochemistry. He can be reached at arun732003@gmail.com.

Contents

Preface

I take the opportunity to present the first edition of the book on Recent Trends in Cardiovascular Risks with the support of InTech publishers. I thank the publisher for giving me the opportunity to work with them as an editor for this book. This book enthralls on the recent trends of cardiovascular risks, which would be fruitful to readers, researchers, and clinicians in health sciences.

The authors of this book are leading researchers in the field. Most of the cardiovascular risks are widely known, but due to changing trends based on lifestyle and geographical variance, from developing to developed countries, the risks vary. We have tried to compile the risks as a whole so that the readers can benefit from going through the chapters of the book.

I have arranged the chapters based on the priority index, and I hope that this book will have a large audience and will be appreciated by readers. I shall look forward for valuable comments and fruitful suggestions from all readers of medical and health science fraternity, including researchers, for further improvement of the book.

Lastly, I am indebted to InTech publishers for giving me the opportunity to edit this book and all authors whose impeccable contributions where brought out in this new edition of book.

Dr. Arun Kumar
Professor and Head
Department of Biochemistry
Krishna Mohan Medical College and Hospital
Mathura, India

Chapter 1

Introductory Chapter: Recent Trends in Cardiovascular Risk Factors

Arun Kumar

Additional information is available at the end of the chapter

http://dx.doi.org/10.5772/intechopen.69159

We are happy to bring out this new book entitled 'Recent trends in Cardiovascular Risks' which is written by scientifically accredited authors across the globe. The primary and secondary preventions are the effective measures for reducing premature mortality. In context to developed countries, there are five existing modifiable risk factors, namely high blood pressure, high cholesterol, tobacco use-smoking, diabetes mellitus and obesity which constitutes approximately one-third of all CVD cases [1]. Of which highly preventable risk factors such as high blood pressure, obesity and smoking are related to premature mortality and morbidity from cardiovascular disease (CVD) [2]. The modifiable risk factors, namely smoking, obesity and lack of physical activity, account to 36%, 20% and 7–12% of coronary artery disease, respectively [3].

1. Scenario of Cardiovascular Disease

The incidence of AMI is drastically increasing in major developing countries, and it is noticed even in rural population, which has become a potential threat [4]. Other modifiable risk factors include low socioeconomic status, alcohol use, mental ill-health, psychosocial stress and left ventricular hypertrophy. Among the nonmodifiable risk factors are advancing age, heredity or family history, gender, ethnicity or race (**Figure 1**) [5]. To reduce the global burden of mortality from CVD, we need to refine our strategic goals and intervention programs. While we find the global population is expected to rise by almost 20% from 6.7 billion to 8.1 billion by 2030, the crude death rate still remains stable around 8.4 deaths/thousand [1]. Cardiovascular diseases were once thought to be the disease of the rich and affluent class of people, but now it is more visible among the poor as well. Conventional cardiovascular risk is attributed to lifestyle changes and altered metabolic activity.

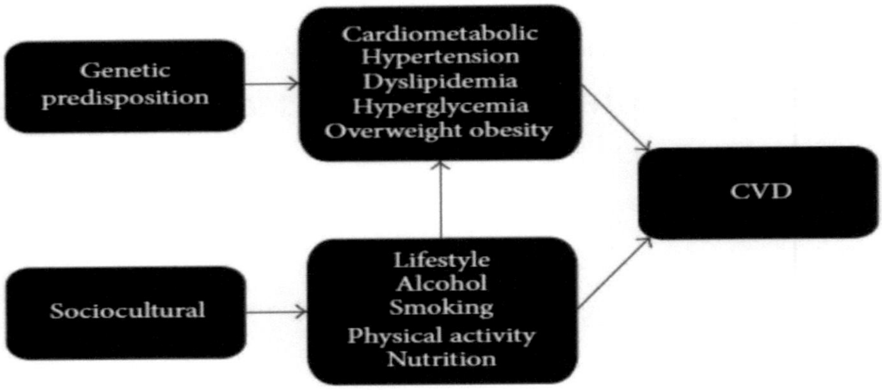

Figure 1. Causative pathways for CVD.

2. Changing Trends of Cardiovascular Risks

The most common emerging trends in cardiovascular risk factors include altered lipid profile, coronary artery calcium score, lipoprotein (a), apolipoproteins, homocysteine, thrombosis markers like fibrinogen, plasminogen activator inhibitor-1, carotid intima-media thickness, genotypic variations, nonalcoholic fatty liver disease, C-reactive protein, platelets and birth weight levels [6].

These diseases not only affect the well being, but can also dampen the economic growth of the country due to enormous healthcare expenditure associated with decreased productivity. Even though abundance curative cares are available in urban areas, this alone cannot suffice the problem of CVDs. The need of the hour is to focus on its prevention and palliative care along with its early diagnosis, and management as it is not the sole responsibility of the health care providers alone can tackle this problem.

3. Awareness is a must among mass

There is an urgent need for all of us to change our lifestyle through positive and negative reinforcements. In rural areas, we need to adopt start-ups, to create awareness among common people so that the disease can be cured at the grassroot level. Through coordination and collaboration with health care sectors including the government and pharmaceutical companies, the awareness can be generated and the risk can be identified.

4. Contents of the book in brief

In this book, we delineate the various risk factors and the current trends of cardiovascular risk factors. This book emphasizes on various issues which are alarming and are potential threats for cardiovascular risk. The overall risk assessment of cardiovascular disease using multivariate scores in developing countries is one of the approaches. This approach is likely to assure that limited resource in developing countries be allocated to those who need it most. The clear justification for cardiovascular risk assessment is crucial for policy decision on the implementation of such a strategy. While many developing countries solely described estimated cardiovascular risk by applying existing CVD risk scores to their population's cross-sectional risk factor data, a number of countries have validated and recalibrated existing risk scores and only a few have developed a new risk score specific to their populations [7]. To enhance the adoption of such a policy in developing countries, an additional strategy by the WHO and International Society of Hypertension was developed by deriving both laboratory- and nonlaboratory-based CVD risk prediction charts for low- and medium-resource settings in countries in different WHO subregions. Significant researches have suggested that a vascular segment gives us a clue of atherosclerotic lesions, namely endothelial dysfunctions, macrophage activation, cellular proliferation and thrombosis, and they respond differently on medication [8]. Therapeutic approach of the atherogenic dyslipidemia imposes the correlation with proatherogenic individual tendencies in order to correct the further risks [9]. Cardiovascular disease appears in coronary arteries when the atherosclerotic lesions evolve from an initial accumulation of isolated foam cells in the arterial intima to fatty streaks, followed by the accumulation of cholesterol deposits and atheroma formation [10]. Cardiovascular disease may have their origin in the intrauterine life, but also a low birth weight and an extremely rich diet increase the risk of obesity and a specific metabolic syndrome in adults [11]. Its incidence and mortality is very low in reproductive age women, but it increases with age [12]. Estradiol (E2) reduces the development of the early atherosclerotic lesions, in some measure, by its effects on the lipid metabolism, with a reduction of the lipid deposits from the intima [13].

5. Facts based on Epidemiological studies

World Health Organization (WHO) conducted numerous studies regarding the mortality due to myocardial infarction, stroke and venous thromboembolism in many countries across the world. Epidemiological studies revealed an increased incidence of myocardial infarction approximately five times higher in individuals between the ages of 40 and 60 years old [14]. Hormonal contraceptives, pregnancy and polycystic ovary syndrome in young women and menopause in older women are directly linked with cardiovascular diseases [15]. Polycystic ovary syndrome should be seen as a metabolic disease, with a high risk in developing diabetes mellitus type 2 and different cardiovascular disease, and is less frequent in women in reproductive age. Another extremely important risk factor involved in women atherosclerosis is heredity. Diabetes mellitus induces hypercholesterolemia and in consequence an increase in predisposition for atherosclerosis in both male and female. The incidence of the myocardial infarction is two times higher at patients with diabetes mellitus compared to patients without diabetes.

6. Metabolic Syndrome an emerging threat

In the last few years, the criteria for metabolic syndrome have been reviewed: abdominal obesity, increased serum cholesterol, high blood pressure, insulin resistance with or without impaired glucose tolerance, pro-inflammatory status, a high level of C-reactive protein and a pro-thrombotic status with a high plasmatic fibrinogen and coagulation factors level [16]. Morphological and experimental studies have demonstrated connections between hyperlipidemia, especially hypercholesterolemia, and atherosclerosis, in both women and men. The content of the atheroma plaque, which is made of cholesterol and cholesterol esters, the structure of the foam cells and the experimental production of atherosclerosis by a high-fat diet have been initial arguments for the implication of lipids in atherosclerosis genesis. Cholesterol and triglycerides are the lipids with the highest impact for atherosclerosis and ischemic cardiomyopathy.

HDL-cholesterol has anti-inflammatory, antioxidant and antithrombotic properties that contribute to the improvement of the endothelial function and atherosclerosis inhibition [17]. Therefore, as the HDL-cholesterol level is higher, the risk of developing atherosclerosis lowers. The physical exercises and moderate consume of ethanol increase the HDL-cholesterol level, while the obesity and smoking are decreasing it [18]. High cholesterol diets or saturated fats, like the ones from the butter, animal fats and yolk, increase the level of the plasmatic cholesterol, while the diets poor in cholesterol and in polyunsaturated fats decrease it.

7. Hypertension as a risk

High blood pressure is a condition characterized by an increase of the systolic value over 140 mmHg and of the diastolic value over 90 mmHg, being a major risk factor for atherosclerosis at all ages, females being less affected. Decreased arterial compliance has a high predictive value for cardiovascular events, so its evaluation becomes an important objective in investigating the arterial function.

Recent studies have shown that smoking is the most important adjustable risk factor in women and men under 40 years old with acute coronary syndrome, being observed in mostly equal parts on those with normal coronary arteries and on those with lesions on one or more coronary arteries.

8. Homocystinuria a silent killer

Patients with homocystinuria, which is a congenital metabolic disorder, characterized by elevated levels of circulating homocysteine (>100 μmol/L) and urinary homocysteine, present an early vascular injury [19]. Clinical and epidemiological studies revealed a connection between the serum levels of homocysteine and peripheral vascular disease, coronary artery disease, stroke and venous thrombosis, meaning that a high concentration of homocysteine is associated with the progression of the atherosclerosis [20].

9. Diabetes and Cardiovascular Disease

Diabetes is now considered as a major and growing health problem worldwide. It causes a considerable amount of disability, premature mortality, loss of productivity and increased demands on health care facilities [21]. According to the World Health Organization, 1 in 20 death is attributable to diabetes, 8700 deaths every day and 6 deaths every minute [22]. Cardiovascular disease is the major cause of morbidity and mortality in people with diabetes, and coronary heart disease is the most common cause of death among people with type 2 diabetes. People with diabetes are two to four times more likely to develop CVD compared with people without the condition [23].

10. Ferritin as an additional risk

Serum ferritin is the main marker of iron status, and hepcidin is the key regulator of iron metabolism, but both are increased in inflammation states; thus, their relationship with pathological processes should be studied with caution. Iron deficiency with severe anemia has been also related to oxidative stress as iron is involved in several enzymatic antioxidant systems. Most studies deal with the association between iron deposition in tissues and cardiovascular risk, while decreased iron status is predominantly related to protection against atherosclerosis and coronary heart disease [24].

So concluding the contents of the book, it focuses on the overall emerging risks in developing and developed countries. We hope that this book would create awareness among mass and also in scientific community across the globe. We tried to bring out and cover most of the recent trends of cardiovascular risks which is prevalent among the society which we tend to condone. It is now high time we look upon ourselves and make resolutions to decrease the existing risks factors which we are on. It is never too late to implement than to overlook. We wish to get the notes and feedback from our readers and rejoice the success of launching this book.

Author details

Arun Kumar

Address all correspondence to: arun732003@gmail.com

Department of Biochemistry, Krishna Mohan Medical College and Hospital, Pali Dungra, Mathura Uttar Pradesh (West), India

References

[1] Kumar A. Changing trends of cardiovascular risk factors among Indians: A review of emerging risks. Asian Pacific Journal of Tropical Biomedicine. 2014;**4**(12):1001-1008. DOI: 10.12980/APJTB.4.201414B401

[2] American Heart Association (n.d.). Risk Factors and Coronary Heart Disease and Stroke. Available from: http://americaheart.org/presenter.jhtml?identifieer=539 [Accessed: September 10, 2006]

[3] Kokkinos P, Sheriff H, Kheirbek R. Physical inactivity and mortality risk. Cardiology Research and Practice. 2011;**2011**:924945

[4] Gaziano TA, Bitton A, Anand S, Abrahams-Gessel S, Murphy A. Growing epidemic of coronary heart disease in low- and middle-income countries. Current Problems in Cardiology. 2010;**35**(2):72-115

[5] Booth FW, Roberts CK, Laye MJ. Lack of exercise is a major cause of chronic diseases. Comprehensive Physiology. 2012;**2**(2):1143-1211

[6] Gupta S, Gudapati R, Gaurav K, Bhise M. Emerging risk factors for cardiovascular diseases: Indian context. Indian Journal of Endocrinology and Metabolism [serial online]. 2013;**17**:806-814. Available from: http://www.ijem.in/text.asp?2013/17/5/806/117212 [Accessed: April 7, 2017]

[7] Damen JAAG, Hooft L, Schuit E, Debray TPA, Collins GS, Tzoulaki I, Lassale CM, Siontis GCM, Chiocchia V, Roberts C, Schlüssel MM, Gerry S, Black JA, Heus P, van der Schouw YT, Peelen LM, Moons KGM. Prediction models for cardiovascular disease risk in the general population: Systematic review. British Medical Journal. 2016;**353**:i2416. DOI: 10.1136/bmj.i2416

[8] Roberts CK, Hevener AL, Barnard RJ. Metabolic syndrome and insulin resistance: Underlying causes and modification by exercise training. Comprehensive Physiology. 2013;**3**(1):1-58. DOI: 10.1002/cphy.c110062

[9] Bosomworth NJ. Approach to identifying and managing atherogenic dyslipidemia. Canadian Family Physician. 2013;**59**(11):1169-1180

[10] Singh RB, Mengi SA, Xu Y-J, Arneja AS, Dhalla NS. Pathogenesis of atherosclerosis: A multifactorial process. Experimental & Clinical Cardiology. 2002;**7**(1):40-53

[11] Calkins K, Devaskar SU. Fetal origins of adult disease. Current Problems in Pediatric and Adolescent Health Care. 2011;**41**(6):158-176. DOI: 10.1016/j.cppeds.2011.01.001

[12] Farley TM, Collins J, Schlesselman JJ. Hormonal contraception and risk of cardiovascular disease. An international perspective. Contraception. 1998;**57**(3):211-230

[13] Reslan OM, Khalil RA. Vascular effects of estrogenic menopausal hormone therapy. Reviews on Recent Clinical Trials. 2012;**7**(1):47-70

[14] Gabriel SE, Michaud K. Epidemiological studies in incidence, prevalence, mortality, and comorbidity of the rheumatic diseases. Arthritis Research & Therapy. 2009;**11**(3):229. DOI: 10.1186/ar2669

[15] ESHRE Capri Workshop Group. Hormones and cardiovascular health in women. Human Reproduction Update. 2006;**12**(5):483-497 [Epub: June 28, 2006]

[16] Kaur J. A comprehensive review on metabolic syndrome. Cardiology Research and Practice. 2014;**2014**:943162. DOI: 10.1155/2014/943162

[17] Besler C, Lüscher TF, Landmesser U. Molecular mechanisms of vascular effects of high-density lipoprotein: Alterations in cardiovascular disease. EMBO Molecular Medicine. 2012;**4**(4):251-268. DOI: 10.1002/emmm.201200224

[18] Buttar HS, Li T, Ravi N. Prevention of cardiovascular diseases: Role of exercise, dietary interventions, obesity and smoking cessation. Experimental & Clinical Cardiology. 2005; **10**(4):229-249

[19] Eldibany MM, Caprini JA. Hyperhomocysteinemia and thrombosis: An overview. Archives of Pathology & Laboratory Medicine. 2007;**131**(6):872-884

[20] Ganguly P, Alam SF. Role of homocysteine in the development of cardiovascular disease. Nutrition Journal. 2015;**14**:6. DOI: 10.1186/1475-2891-14-6

[21] Lunenfeld B, Stratton P. The clinical consequences of an ageing world and preventive strategies. Best Practice & Research: Clinical Obstetrics & Gynaecology. 2013;**27**(5):643-659. DOI: 10.1016/j.bpobgyn.2013.02.005

[22] Roger VL, Go AS, Lloyd-Jones DM, Adams RJ, Berry JD, Brown TM, Carnethon MR, Dai S, de Simone G, Ford ES, Fox CS, Fullerton HJ, Gillespie C, Greenlund KJ, Hailpern SM, Heit JA, Ho PM, Howard VJ, Kissela BM, Kittner SJ, Lackland DT, Lichtman JH, Lisabeth LD, Makuc DM, Marcus GM, Marelli A, Matchar DB, McDermott MM, Meigs JB, Moy CS, Mozaffarian D, Mussolino ME, Nichol G, Paynter NP, Rosamond WD, Sorlie PD, Stafford RS, Turan TN, Turner MB, Wong ND, Wylie-Rosett J. Heart disease and stroke statistics—2011 update: A report from the American Heart Association. Circulation. 2011;**123**(4):e18-e209. DOI: 10.1161/CIR.0b013e3182009701 [Published online: December 15, 2010]

[23] Martín-Timón I, Sevillano-Collantes C, Segura-Galindo A, del Cañizo-Gómez FJ. Type 2 diabetes and cardiovascular disease: Have all risk factors the same strength? World Journal of Diabetes. 2014;**5**(4):444-470

[24] Basuli D, Stevens RG, Torti FM, Torti SV. Epidemiological associations between iron and cardiovascular disease and diabetes. Frontiers in Pharmacology. 2014;**5**:117

Chapter 2

Cardiovascular Risk Factors and its Transition: An Ongoing Cohort Study in Chinese Kazakhs

Jingmei Jiang, Mingtao Zhang, Lei Hou, Wei Han,
Yong Tang, Shaohua Liang and Weizhi Wang

Additional information is available at the end of the chapter

http://dx.doi.org/10.5772/intechopen.69347

Abstract

Studies on the prevalence of risk factors and the incidence for cardiovascular diseases (CVDs) are limited in Kazakh population. By incorporating nomads, farmers, and urban residents, aged 30 years or older, in a cohort study, we investigated the characteristics of cardiovascular risk factors and their temporal trends that arose from the urbanization and subsequent changes in the lifestyle in a Kazakh population with 1668 participants. We used current guidelines and the monitoring trends and determinants in cardiovascular disease (MONICA) standard to define cardiovascular events. Kazakhs had a high prevalence rate of hypertension (45.3%), and this prevalence was much higher than the national average in China. Prevalence of two or more risk factors was highest among urban people and lowest among nomads. Urban residents have the highest prevalence of hypercholesterolemia and obesity compared with farmers and nomads. However, unlike other studies, our data indicate that young men had the highest prevalence of dyslipidemia, and it decreased significantly thereafter. Crude rates of incidence and mortality for acute cardiovascular events were 742 and 194 per 100,000 people, respectively; the standardized rates were 926 and 272 per 100,000 people, respectively. The findings from this study demonstrate the pervasive burden of cardiovascular risk factors and the related acute cardiovascular events in Kazakhs, particularly BP in Kazakh nomads.

Keywords: cardiovascular disease, risk factor, cohort, Chinese Kazakhs, registries

1. Introduction

Cardiovascular diseases (CVDs), such as coronary artery disease and stroke, are the major cause of morbidity, mortality, and health expenses in China and worldwide. According to the large international INTERHEART study (1990–2010), the so-called conventional risk factors, such as hypertension, abnormal serum cholesterol, diabetes mellitus, smoking, and obesity, contributed to approximately 90% of CVDs [1, 2]. In China, existing researches on cardiovascular risk factors are largely related to Han people (the largest ethnic group among 56 ethnic groups of China); comprehensive data on cardiovascular risk factors are limited in other minority groups, such as Kazakh people. Knowing the pattern of cardiovascular risk factors among the minority groups is important not only for predicting the future situation of the epidemic and planning relevant policies for prevention and control of CVDs but also for providing new etiological insights through their juxtaposition to known variations in disease patterns.

The Kazakh is a typical transnational ethnic group with a Eurasian lineage. It is the main ethnic group in Kazakhstan and represents a sizable ethnic minority in China and Russia. There are approximately 1.25 million Kazakh people in China, who mainly (96%) live in the Northern Xinjiang Uygur Autonomous region, as a part of the ancient Silk Road. For thousands of years, China's Kazakh people have mainly been active in raising livestock on the prairie grasslands. With urbanization, modern Kazakh people have naturally formed three different subgroups with different occupational backgrounds, that is, nomads following the traditional mode of year-round migration, farmers settling and engaging in agriculture, and urban people transferring to cities with an increased educational level and economic status. In this chapter, we tried to tell a study-based Kazakh story for readers. This study was conducted in Altay, Northern Xinjiang, and China, and we called it as the "China Altay Kazakh Heart Study (CAKH)" study. Its aim was to investigate whether factors such as environmental and occupational changes have an influence on the risk factors and sequent events of CVDs and to quantify morbidity and mortality of CVDs prospectively among Kazakh people.

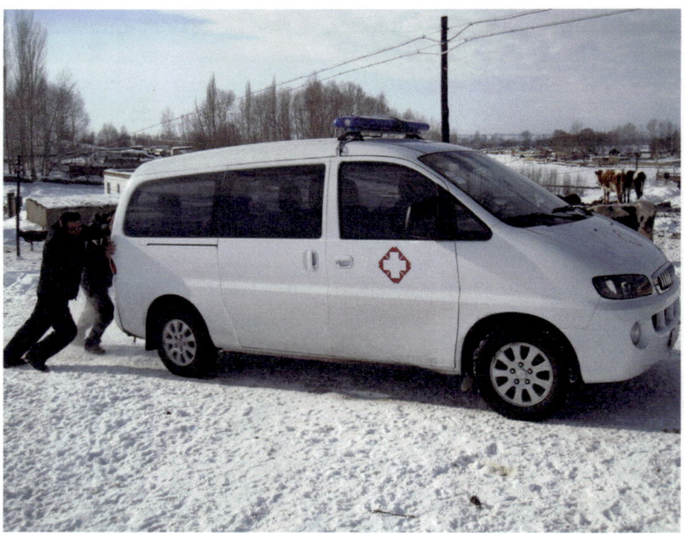

http://dx.doi.org/10.5772/intechopen.69347

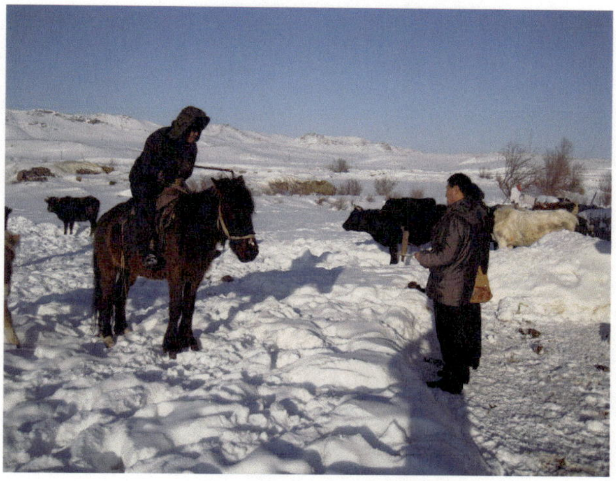

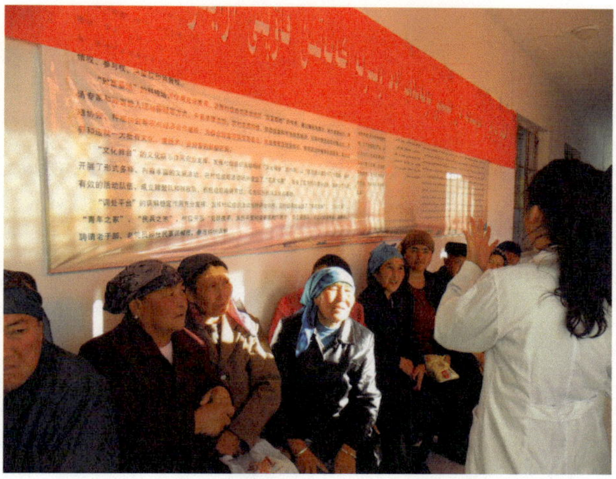

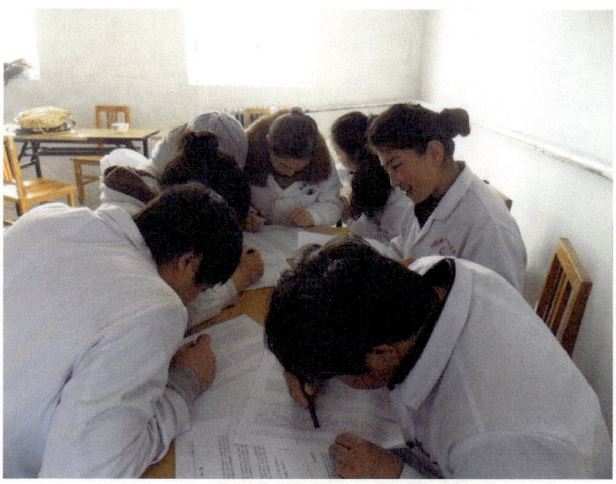

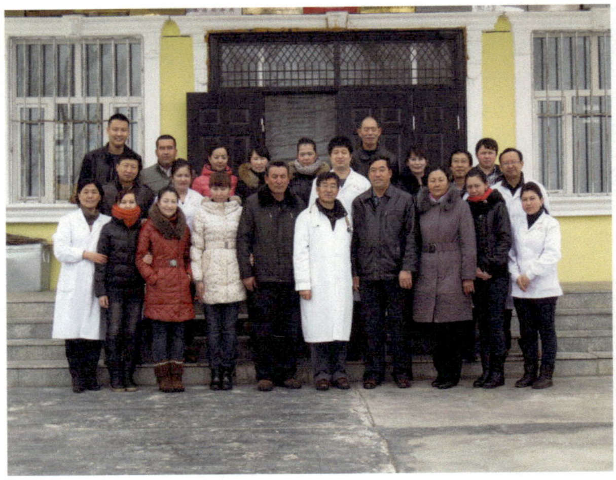

2. Methods

2.1. Study participants

The CAKH study was initiated in 2012 with a community-based design. Hong Dun town, the study base, is located in the urban-rural fringe of Altay county-level city. As shown in **Figure 1**, 12 Kazakh-based administrative villages and one township office, which almost covered all citizens of this town, were included in this study after excluding villages with less

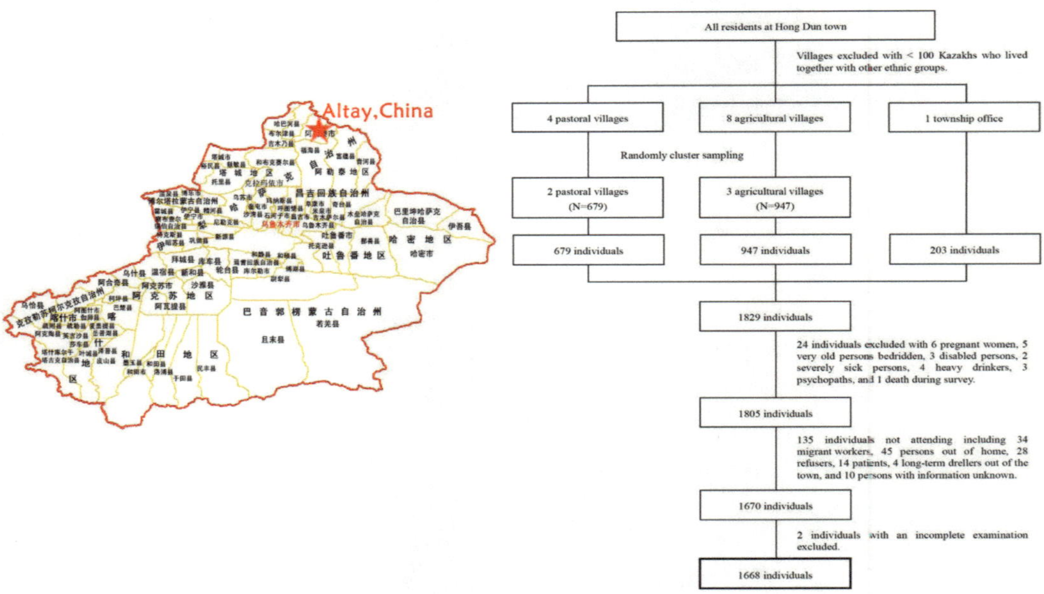

Figure 1. Flow chart of recruitment of participants (also see our previous publication [3]).

than 100 Kazakh individuals who lived together with other ethnic groups. The advantages of Hong Dun town as the study base are that there is a high concentration of Kazakh people, its economic development is representative of the Altay region (one of residence places of Chinese Kazakh with the highest population density), and it includes three natural occupational groups of the Kazakh people, that is, complete nomadic village, farming village, and downtown populations. Using the population census of the area as our sampling frame, a stratified random cluster sampling method was used to select study subjects based on their occupational backgrounds. Samples of potential participants were drawn from two out of four villages characterized by animal husbandry and three out of eight agricultural villages. The entire Kazakh staff affiliated to the township office was recruited into the urban sample. Thus, the final baseline population consisted of five administrative villages (six natural villages) and the downtown professional people, covering 58.4% of the total qualified Kazakh population of the study base of the CAKH study.

All participants included were required to be 30 years of age or older, with at least three generations living in the same region, and were required to have no history of intermarriage. Examinations were performed in the morning, and the elderly or people in remote places were picked up by buses to maximize the participation rate. A participant who had biological Kazakh parents and Kazakh paternal/maternal biological grandparents was considered as a Kazakh. Pregnant women, bedridden persons aged 80 years or older, disabled persons, or persons with severe diseases determined by the investigators were excluded. About 1805 people participated in the survey and 1668 people were completed the survey (see **Figure 1**). This represented 92.4% compliance; specifically, 94.4% (637/675) from pastoral villages, 90.2% (838/929) from agricultural villages, and 96.0% (193/201) from the township office. Their distribution in each sampling unit is displayed in **Table 1**. The overall response rate for completing both the survey and the physical examination was 92.4% (94.4% for pastoral villages, 90.2% for agricultural villages, and 96.0% for urban professional workers). We confirmed that all institutional and governmental regulations concerning the ethical use of human volunteers were followed for this study, which was approved by the Ethical Committees of Chinese Academy of Medical Sciences and Peking Union Medical College.

Village or township office	Occupation	Person number	Men (%)	Age (years, mean (SD))
Kesirjia	Nomads	147	50.3	43.8 (10.4)
Tarstark	Nomads	212	45.8	47.2 (12.7)
Bitiworg	Nomads	278	46.0	47.7 (12.8)
Wutubulak	Farmers	193	47.0	47.9 (12.3)
Sarkamus	Farmers	377	50.9	48.1 (13.3)
Duolart	Farmers	270	47.6	46.3 (12.3)
Township office	Urban people	191	36.3	41.8 (8.9)

Kesirjia and Tarstark are natural villages both affiliated to one administrative village.

Table 1. Participants enrolled in each sampling unit.

2.2. Questionnaire survey

The baseline investigation of the CAKH study was conducted from October 2012 to February 2013 when all nomads would return to their 'home in winter;' this time period included the most important Kazakh holiday, that is, the Corban Festival.

A unified questionnaire was administered through face-to-face interviews conducted by trained and qualified Kazakh medical college students. Information included demographic factors, socioeconomic status (SES) (educational level, marital status, and annual household income), cigarette smoking, alcohol consumption, and information about personal or family history of selected conditions. In addition, based on the characteristics of the Kazakh people, we set up a series of questions about dietary habits. For example, we set four possible responses for vegetable and fruit intake, each category ranging from never or less than once per week to seven or more times per week; we also asked the respondent to give the name and type of the fruit and vegetables they ate. Dietary habits included self-reported volumes of milk-tea consumed (a kind of tea with milk and salt) as well as frequency of consumption of air-dried meats (a kind of meat with salt used as the preservative). Consumption of fruit and vegetables was incorporated into the questionnaire and was coded as more than seven times per week, four to six times per week, one to three times per week, less than once a week, or no fruit and vegetables used.

2.3. Physical examination

Physical examinations included weight, height, and waist circumference measurements, and body mass index (BMI) was calculated as body weight (kg) divided by height (m^2). We used an appropriate arm cuff and a mercury column sphygmomanometer to measure BPs of the left arm in the supine position. Before measurements, a resting period of at least 10 min was required. The mean of two readings or three readings, if there was a difference of more than 5 mmHg between the initial readings, was taken as BP values for the final analysis [4]. A standard 12-lead electrocardiogram (ECG) was conducted for each participant.

2.4. Laboratory measurements

A venous blood sample and a second urine sample after waking were collected from each participant after an overnight fast of at least 10 h, and plasma was immediately separated. All the samples were tested in the central laboratory of the People's Hospital of Altay Prefecture. Total cholesterol (TC), triglycerides (TG), fasting blood glucose (FBG), and creatinine were measured by a standard enzymatic method. Direct determination of concentrations of high-density lipoprotein cholesterol (HDL-C) and low-density lipoprotein cholesterol (LDL-C) were simultaneously performed. Sodium intake was assessed by urinary sodium excretion from the second urine sample after waking, urinary creatinine concentration, and 24-h urinary creatinine excreted as estimated from height, body weight, and age, as shown in **Table 2** [5]. Daily salt intake was estimated based on a calculation of 24-h urinary sodium excretion on the assumption that all sodium ingested was in the form of sodium chloride, with each 43 mmol of sodium being approximately equivalent to 2.5 g of salt (sodium chloride). Chemistry measurements were made using a Beckman Coulter AU2700 Clinical Chemistry Analyzer (Brea, CA, USA). Electrolytes were measured using a Caretium XI-921 CT Electrolyte Analyzer (Shenzhen, China).

24-h Na excretion (mmol/day) = $16.3 \times \sqrt{(Na_{SMU}/Cr_{SMU})} \times Pr.UCr_{24}$
Na_{SMU}: Na concentration in second urine sample after waking (mEq/L)
Cr_{SMU}: Cr concentration in second urine sample after waking (mg/L)
$Pr.UCr_{24}$: estimated 24-h urinary Cr excretion (mg/day)
Male Body weight (kg) × 15.1 + Height (cm) × 7.4 − Age × 12.4 − 80
Female Body weight (kg) × 8.6 + Height (cm) × 5.1 − Age × 4.7 − 75
Cr, creatinine

Table 2. Formula for the estimation of the 24-h Na excretion from the data in the second urine sample after waking and estimated Cr excretion.

2.5. Definition of cardiovascular risk factors

Conventional cardiovascular risk factors were defined based on current national guidelines [6]. Hypertension was defined as a systolic BP (SBP) ≥ 140 mmHg, a diastolic BP (DBP) ≥ 90 mmHg, or both, or the use of antihypertensive medications within the last two weeks [6]. Dyslipidemia was defined as total cholesterol (TC) ≥ 6.22 mmol/L, or LDL-C ≥ 4.14 mmol/L, or HDL-C < 1.04 mmol/L, or TG > 2.26 mmol/L, or receiving cholesterol-lowering medication [7]. Obesity was defined as a BMI ≥ 28.0 (kg/m^2). Diabetes mellitus was defined as fasting blood glucose concentration ≥ 7.0 mmol/L or taking hypoglycemic agents. Current smokers were defined as those who had smoked at least one cigarette each day during the past year [8]. Women who consume one or more alcoholic drinks per day and men who consume two or more alcoholic drinks per day were considered as current alcohol drinkers.

2.6. Collection of acute cardiovascular events

This ongoing prospective cohort study currently completed the first collection of acute cardiovascular events from October 1, 2012 through June 30, 2016 in 1668 participants. The next follow-up is being planned. Acute cardiovascular events included stroke, acute myocardial infarction (AMI), and sudden cardiac death (SCD). Stroke and AMI could be fatal or nonfatal. Stroke events were defined as rapidly developing signs of focal (or global) disturbance of cerebral function lasting 24 hours (unless interrupted by surgery or death) with no apparent nonvascular cause according to the World Health Organization (WHO) MONICA standard [9]. On the basis of the status within 28 days of onset, stroke and AMI events were subdivided into first or recurrent and into fatal or nonfatal. The 2012 universal definition of myocardial infarction was used for AMIs [10]. Considering a factual situation of monitoring cardiovascular diseases, AMIs were classified into definite or possible/insufficient ones particularly for fatal cases according to MONICA standard, with deaths due to chronic coronary heart diseases excluded [9, 11]. An SCD is defined as sudden and unexpected death within an hour of symptom-onset after excluding participants whose sudden deaths were likely due to a known noncardiac cause, such as a large pulmonary embolism that could result in cardiac arrest or malignancy that is not in remission. If unwitnessed, subjects should have been observed alive within 24 hours of their deaths [12]. The WHO's International Classification of Diseases, the

10th revision (ICD-10) was used in this study. The code of I60–I64 was for stroke, including hemorrhagic (I60–I62), ischemic (I63), and nonspecified stroke (I64). The code of cardiac events included I21–I22 for acute myocardial infarction and I46.1 for sudden cardiac death. Information on demographic characteristics, diagnosis such as imaging, markers of myocardial injury, and electrocardiogram, and time of event onset and death was also collected. In addition, for a high quality of registration of acute cardiovascular events, information on all deaths within this period were recorded, such as underlying and direct causes of all deaths, the place and time of death, diagnoses and related evidence, and so on. Discharge records were mainly used to qualify diagnoses, and for patients who did not visit the clinics of local hospitals, any other medical records and inquires by doctors were employed.

Three survey stages for collecting acute cardiovascular events, that is, a hospital-based search and reading of medical records of inpatients in all four local hospitals (i.e., the People's Hospital of Altay Prefecture, the People's Hospital of Altay City, the 16th People's Liberation Army Hospital, and the Kazakh Hospital of Altay), a supplementary registration from village physicians, and a survey for reducing false negatives, were included in this work. On August 10–12, 2016, we visited the departments responsible for medical records in these four hospitals. We searched all files indexed by discharge date, residence, and ICD-10 codes. After excluding some files according to ethnics, names, and age, an expert committee including clinical doctors and public health doctors read medical courses, judged an acute cardiovascular event, and filled an event card out. On August 11, 2016, we trained all related village physicians who were responsible for collecting clues on the occurrence of acute cardiovascular events in selected subjects. On August 15, 2016, these clues were submitted to the expert committee. For patients with a history of hospitalization, a reading of medical records and a judgment for identifying acute cardiovascular events were done; for the ones not hospitalized or whose deaths occurred at home, a detailed inquiry was conducted for the relatives of patients and related village physicians. Also, electronic files of medical insurance were used to search related cases. No loss to follow-up was found. On August 26, 2016, with checking the preliminary results of collection, we found zero events identified in the township office, thereafter a recheck was done by telephone through village physicians.

2.7. Statistical analysis

Initially the distribution of each cardiovascular risk factor was examined among three groups by gender. We calculated the prevalence with 95% confidence intervals for binary variables and means with standard deviations for continuous variables; medians (interquartile range) are presented for triglycerides and fasting blood glucose since these data were positively skewed. All reported values (means, prevalence) were adjusted for age using linear regression or logistic regression models. We assessed trends in educational attainment and economic measures by fitting regression models for each outcome and performing the Wald test on model parameters. The incidence refers to all events, first or recurrent and nonfatal or fatal, within one year per 100,000 people, and mortality rate is the number of fatal events within 28 days per 100,000 people [9]. The incidence and mortality were standardized with the weights from distribution of age and gender in the Sixth National Census of China conducted in 2010. A Chi square test was used to compare difference of groups for

http://dx.doi.org/10.5772/intechopen.69347

qualitative data. All *P*-values were two-sided except *P* trend tests based on nonconditional logistic method, in which one-sided *P* values were used, and a *P*-value < 0.05 was considered statistically significant. All analysis was conducted with the use of SAS 9.2 Version (Institute, Inc., Cary, NC, USA).

3. Results

In general, the farmer group had the highest proportion (50.2%) of the participants and the eldest median age (45; range 30–85 years), followed by the nomad group (the proportion was 38.2% and median age 44; range 30 to 88 years) and the urban group had the lowest participating proportions (11.6%) and the youngest median age (39; range 30 to 78 years). About 24.5% of the participants had a high school education or higher, 88.1% were married and living with a spouse, and 41.2% had annual family income between 10,000 and 40,000 RMB. Basic medical insurance covered almost all of the participants (97.8%). The study population was relatively stable with a mobile population (migrant workers) of 1.9%. The characteristics of the participants in each subgroup by gender are shown in **Table 3**.

	Nomads			**Farmers**			**Urban group**		
	Men	**Women**	**Total**	**Men**	**Women**	**Total**	**Men**	**Women**	**Total**
No.	299	338	637	410	428	838	70	123	193
Age (years, Mean (SD))	46.6 (12.2)	46.6 (12.5)	46.6 (12.3)	46.9 (12.3)	48.3 (13.1)	47.6 (12.7)	43.5 (10.0)	40.8 (8.0)	41.8 (8.9)
Education (years, mean (SD))									
≤Primary school	124 (41.6)	138 (41.1)	262 (41.3)	114 (28.0)	125 (29.3)	239 (28.7)	1 (1.4)	1 (0.8)	2 (1.0)
Middle school	145 (48.7)	164 (48.8)	309 (48.7)	227 (55.8)	200 (46.8)	427 (51.2)	6 (8.6)	10 (8.1)	16 (8.3)
High school or above	29 (9.7)	34 (10.1)	63 (9.9)	66 (12.2)	102 (23.9)	168 (20.1)	63 (90.0)	112 (91.1)	175 (90.7)
Marital status									
Married	257 (89.6)	287 (85.4)	554 (87.4)	362 (88.9)	370 (86.7)	732 (87.8)	68 (97.1)	110 (89.4)	178 (92.23)
Other*	31 (10.4)	49 (14.6)	80 (12.6)	45 (11.1)	57 (13.4)	102 (12.2)	2 (2.9)	13 (10.6)	15 (7.8)
Annual family income (RMB)									
<10 000	163 (54.9)	192 (57.5)	355 (56.3)	228 (56.2)	259 (61.7)	487 (59.0)	11 (15.7)	24 (19.5)	35 (18.1)
10 000–40 000	117 (39.4)	132 (39.5)	249 (39.5)	163 (40.2)	150 (35.7)	313 (37.9)	45 (64.3)	72 (58.5)	117 (60.6)
≥40 000	17 (5.7)	10 (3.0)	27 (4.3)	15 (3.7)	11 (2.6)	26 (3.2)	14 (24.0)	27 (22.0)	41 (21.2)

	Nomads			Farmers			Urban group		
	Men	Women	Total	Men	Women	Total	Men	Women	Total
Medical insurance									
Yes	295 (99.0)	324 (96.4)	619 (97.6)	399 (98.3)	419 (98.1)	818 (98.2)	69 (98.6)	118 (95.9)	187 (96.9)
No	3 (1.0)	12 (3.6)	15 (2.4)	7 (1.7)	8 (1.9)	15 (1.8)	1 (1.4)	5 (4.1)	6 (3.1)
Go out for work in past year									
Yes	8 (2.7)	2 (0.6)	10 (1.6)	20 (4.9)	5 (1.2)	25 (3.0)	5 (7.1)	5 (4.1)	10 (5.2)
No	285 (95.3)	333 (98.5)	618 (97.0)	381 (93.0)	415 (97.0)	796 (95.0)	64 (91.4)	118 (95.9)	182 (94.3)

*Separated, divorced, or widowed. Data on marital status, annual family income, medical insurance, and going out for work in the past year are person numbers (percents) of participants.

Table 3. Descriptive characteristics for Kazakh participants by occupational background and by gender.

3.1. Distribution of cardiovascular risk factors

Table 4 shows the distribution of cardiovascular risk factors by occupational categories and by gender. We observed a significantly diverse pattern between groups for the risk factor measurements. Nomad men and women had the highest mean levels of SBP and DBP, TC, LDL-C, HDL-C, and FBG, followed by the farmer group, and the urban men and women had the lowest level in most subgroups (all $P < 0.001$). The main exceptions were for BMI and TG level where an opposite trend was observed. Compared with nomads and farmers, urban people, both men and women, had the highest mean level of BMI and TG though there was less statistical significance in the trend in TG level among urban women.

Age-adjusted prevalence of cardiovascular risk factors by occupational backgrounds and by gender is presented in **Figure 2**. The overall prevalence (95% CI) of hypertension was 50.0% (49.0%, 51.1%) among men and ranged from 47.1% (44.3%, 49.9%) (urban men) to 54.2% (52.5%, 55.8%) (nomad men). In women, prevalence of hypertension was 41.1% (39.3%, 42.8%) and ranged from 22.8% (19.2%, 26.3%) (urban women) to 47.0% (44.2%, 49.9%) (nomad women). Nomad group, both men and women, had the highest rates of hypertension (all $P < 0.001$). Overall, 39.4% (38.9%, 39.9%) of men had dyslipidemia; dyslipidemia prevalence ranged from 37.5% (37.2%, 37.7%) (nomad men) to 55.7% (53.9%, 57.5%) (urban men). Overall prevalence of dyslipidemia among women was 24.1% (23.8%, 24.4%), which ranged from 23.4% (22.7–24.0%) (nomad women) to 30.1% (29.7%, 30.4%) (urban women). Urban group, both men and women, had the highest rates of dyslipidemia (all $P < 0.001$). About 26.2% (26.1, 26.3%) of men were obese; prevalence of obesity ranged from 24.4% (24.1%, 24.6%) (farmer men) to 41.4% (40.3%, 42.5%) (urban men). Among women, overall prevalence of obesity was 37.8% (37.3%, 38.2%). Prevalence of obesity was the highest (44.7%) (42.5%, 46.9%) for urban women the lowest 33.7% (32.9%, 34.5%) for nomad women. Urban group, both men and women, had the highest rates of obesity (all $P < 0.001$). Overall, 1.9% (1.8%, 2.0%) of men and 1.2% (1.1%, 1.3%) of women had diabetes mellitus, ranging from 1.2% (1.1%, 1.3%) in farmer men to 2.9% (0.9%, 4.8%) in urban men and from 0.7% (0.6%, 0.8%) in farmer women

	Men				Women			
	Nomad (n=299)	**Farmer (n=410)**	**Urban people (n=70)**	***P* for trend***	**Nomad (n=338)**	**Farmer (n=427)**	**Urban people (n=123)**	***P* for trend***
Mean (SD) SBP (mmHg)	140.8 (23.0)	135.9(20.9)	132.2 (16.7)	0.001	138.2 (27.1)	134.3 (26.1)	125.8 (19.6)	< 0.001
Mean (SD) DBP (mmHg)	88.5 (13.8)	85.3 (12.8)	85.7 (11.8)	0.005	85.3 (14.2)	82.2 (12.8)	81.2 (11.8)	0.001
Mean (SD) BMI (kg/m^2)	25.6 (4.4)	25.5 (4.1)	27.1 (4.6)	0.011	26.5 (5.2)	27.1 (5.1)	27.5 (4.3)	0.085
Mean (SD) TC (mmol/L)	5.40 (0.94)	5.18 (0.94)	5.31 (1.01)	0.009	5.08 (0.91)	4.95 (0.96)	4.60 (0.81)	< 0.001
Mean (SD) LDL-C (mmol/L)	3.27 (0.61)	3.02 (0.60)	3.22 (0.64)	<0.001	3.10 (0.60)	2.92 (0.61)	2.76 (0.50)	< 0.001
Mean (SD) HDL-C (mmol/L)	1.42 (0.42)	1.33 (0.35)	1.26 (0.54)	0.001	1.48 (0.40)	1.43 (0.33)	1.24 (0.29)	< 0.001
Median (IQR) TG (mmol/L)	0.87 (0.62, 1.30)	0.94 (0.71, 1.43)	1.29 (0.91, 2.27)	0.002	0.76 (0.58, 1.03)	0.82 (0.58, 1.11)	0.82 (0.62, 1.10)	0.647
Median (IQR) FBG (mmol/L)	5.34 (5.03, 5.64)	5.24 (4.95, 5.53)	4.98 (4.74, 5.33)	0.026	5.17 (4.89, 5.44)	5.08 (4.78, 5.37)	4.90 (4.64, 5.22)	0.107

*P values were obtained by fitting regression models with risk factors as the outcome and performing Wald tests on model parameters (logistic regression was used for binary variables and linear regression for continuous variables).

SD: standard deviation; IQR: interquartile range; HDL-C: high-density lipoprotein cholesterol; LDL-C: low-density lipoprotein cholesterol; BP: blood pressure.

Table 4. Levels of BP, blood lipid, and fasting blood glucose in Kazakhs of three occupational backgrounds by gender.

to 3.3% (2.0%, 4.5%) in urban women, respectively; urban men and women had the highest diabetes prevalence (all $P < 0.001$). About 55.6% (54.9%, 56.4%) of men were current smokers, with highest prevalence of smoking among urban men (62.9, 61.8–63.9%) and lowest among farmer men (54.2, 53.0–55.4%). Overall, the prevalence of current smoking in women was low (2.6%, 2.5% to 2.7%); the highest prevalence of smoking was 4.4% (4.3%, 4.7%) among nomad women and the lowest was 1.4% (1.3%, 1.5%) among farmer women (all $P < 0.001$). These rates were largely unchanged when standardized to the Kazakh general population in 2010.

Table 5 shows the age- and occupation-adjusted prevalence of cardiovascular risk factors by SES. For men, hypertension was more common in the lower educational attainment (ranged from 55.6 to 44.9% from low to high level) and lower annual family income (ranged from 55.9 to 46.1%) group, whereas dyslipidemia and obesity were more common in the higher educational attainment (from 34.3 to 55.1% for dyslipidemia; 12.2 to 22.8% for obesity) and economic level group (from 37.3 to 44.5% for dyslipidemia; 13.1 to 18.9% for obesity), both showed a significant linear gradient relationship (all $P < 0.01$). Similar to men, hypertension

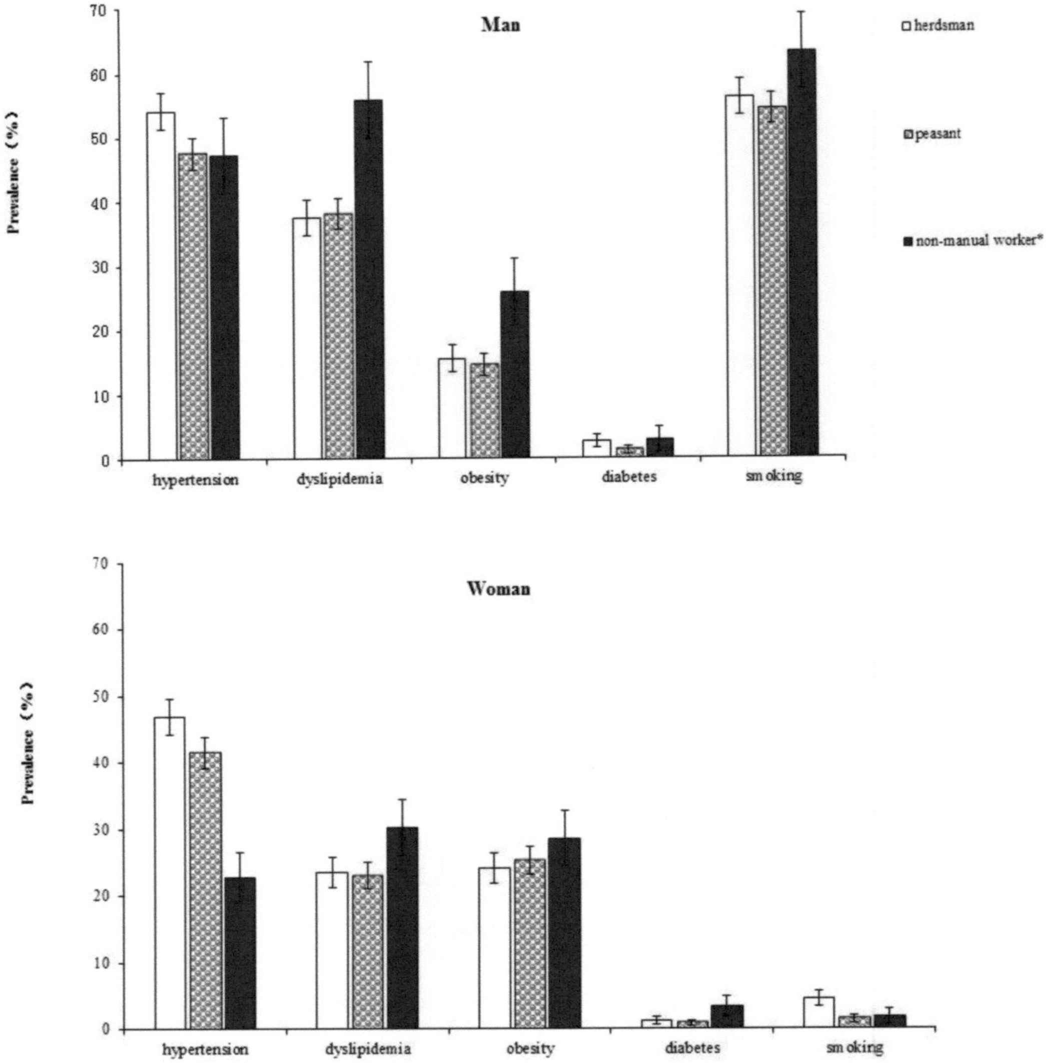

Figure 2. Prevalence of adverse cardiovascular disease risk profiles for all participants by occupational backgrounds and gender. *Risk factors: Hypertension was defined as systolic blood pressure ≥ 140 mm Hg, diastolic blood pressure ≥ 90 mm Hg, or receiving treatment; Dyslipidemia was defined as total cholesterol (TC) ≥ 6.22 mmol/L, or LDL cholesterol ≥ 4.14 mmol/L, or HDL cholesterol < 1.04 mmol/L, or TG >1.70mmol; Obesity was defined as a body mass index ≥ 28 kg/m^2; Diabetes mellitus was defined as fasting blood glucose concentration ≥ 7.0 mmol/L or take hypoglycemic agents; Smoking was defined as currently smoking cigarettes. Values were adjusted for age. Error bars indicate 95% CIs (also see our previous publication [12]).

in women was found to be more common in lower educational level and lower annual family income group (the prevalence from 59.1 to 25.0% following an increasing educational level; from 51.8 to 37.8% following an increasing annual family income level, all $P < 0.001$), but there was no such trend in the distribution of dyslipidemia with SES. There was no significant trend in other risk factors' distribution with regard to the level of SES.

http://dx.doi.org/10.5772/intechopen.69347

	Men's educational level †				Women's educational level †			
	Low (n=239)	**Middle (n=378)**	**High (n=158)**	**P for trend**	**Low (n=338)**	**Middle (n=427)**	**High (n=123)**	**P for trend**
Hypertension (%)	55.6 (49.4, 61.9)	48.7 (43.6, 53.7)	44.9 (37.2, 52.7)	0.030	59.1 (53.2, 65.0)	38.8 (33.8,43.7)	25.0 (19.6, 30.4)	<0.001
Dyslipidemia (%)	34.3 (28.3, 40.3)	36.2 (31.4, 41.1)	55.1 (47.3, 62.8)	< 0.001	26.9 (21.5, 32.2)	23.8 (19.5, 28.1)	21.8 (16.6, 26.9)	0.175
Obesity (%)	12.2 (8.1, 16.4)	15.3 (11.7, 19.0)	22.8 (16.2, 26.3)	0.007	26.7 (21.4, 32.0)	25.9 (21.5, 30.4)	22.6 (17.4, 27.8)	0.298
Diabetes (%)	1.3 (0.0, 2.7)	2.6 (1.0, 4.3)	1.3 (0.5, 3.0)	0.834	1.1 (0.0, 2.4)	1.3 (0.2, 2.5)	1.2 (0.0, 2.6)	0.937
Smoking (%)	50.2 (43.9, 56.5)	59.0 (54.0, 64.0)	56.3 (48.6, 64.1)	0.148	1.9 (0.2, 3.5)	3.7 (1.8, 5.7)	1.6 (0.0, 3.2)	0.871
	Men's annual family income ‡				Women's annual family income‡			
	Low (n=299)	Middle (n=410)	High (n=70)	*P*	Low (n=338)	Middle (n=427)	High (n=123)	*P*
Hypertension (%)	55.0 (47.5, 62.5)	53.2 (46.8, 59.6)	46.1 (41.0, 51.2)	0.034	51.8 (44.2, 59.4)	38.5 (33.1, 43.9)	37.8 (33.1, 42.6)	0.006
Dyslipidemia (%)	37.3 (30.0, 44.6)	33.5 (27.4, 39.5)	44.5 (39.4, 49.5)	0.041	25.3 (18.7, 31.9)	20.7 (16.2, 25.2)	25.9 (21.6, 30.2)	0.567
Obesity (%)	13.1 (8.0, 18.2)	13.4 (9.0, 17.7)	18.9 (14.9, 22.8)	0.053	27.1 (20.3, 33.9)	23.0 (18.3, 27.7)	26.0 (21.7, 30.3)	0.999
Diabetes (%)	2.4 (0.1, 4.7)	3.0 (0.8, 5.2)	1.1 (0.0, 2.1)	0.198	1.2 (0.0, 2.9)	1.0 (0.0, 2.1)	1.5 (0.3, 2.7)	0.677
Smoking (%)	58.0 (50.5, 65.4)	56.7 (50.3, 63.0)	54.2 (49.1, 59.2)	0.380	2.4 (0.1, 4.7)	2.9 (1.0, 4.8)	2.2 (0.8, 3.7)	0.793

Percents (95% CIs) were adjusted for age and occupational background.

†Educational level was defined as: low ≤ primary school middle: middle school; high: high school or above.

‡Annual family income (RMB) was defined as: low: < 10,000; middle: 10,000–40, 000; and high: ≥ 40,000(RMB).

Table 5. The prevalence of CVD risk factors by socioeconomic position and by gender among Kazakh participants.

Overall, 33.2% of men had a level of any one major risk factor only (most commonly smoke, 50.8%); 35.3% and 21.1% of men had any 2 only or 3 or more risk factors, as shown in **Figure 3**. Prevalence of 3 or more risk factors was highest among urban men (30.0%) and lowest among nomad men (20.1%) ($P < 0.001$). Among women, 33.3% had one risk factor only (most commonly hypertension, 44.3%); 24.3% and 8.1% had any 2, 3, or more risk factors. Prevalence of three or more risk factors was the highest among urban women (11.4%) and lowest among nomad women (6.5%) ($P < 0.001$). A significantly higher proportion ($P < 0.001$) of men than women had three or more risk factors. Prevalence of three or more risk factors was significantly higher ($P < 0.001$) with lower annual family income and lower education attainment (women only). The respective prevalence in men and women ranged from 48.9% and 52.9% for low family income group to 6.1% and 7.4% for high level family income group; and the respective prevalence ranged from 44.4 to 22.2% for women from low to high level of education ($P < 0.001$), but this trend revealed opposite for men with 20.7 and 28.7% from low to high level of education ($P < 0.05$).

In addition, we estimated 24-h salt intake of 17.6 ± 14.2 g/d in this population. This value was 17.6 (16.8), 16.9 (12.7), and 20.7 (9.8) g/d in these three occupational groups, respectively. Though high dietary salt intake was not associated with occupational background, a significant association of salt intake with BP level was observed among 1445 participants (86.6%) who did not take antihypertensive medication, as shown in **Figure 4**. This association on

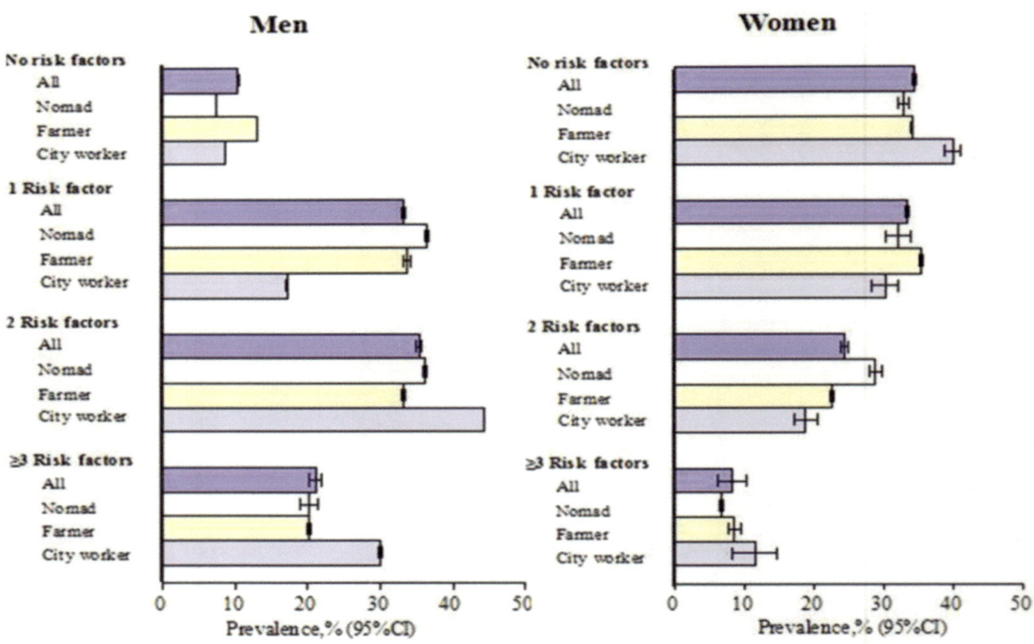

Figure 3. Comparison of profiles of risk factors by occupational backgrounds in men and women (also see our previous publication [12]).

http://dx.doi.org/10.5772/intechopen.69347

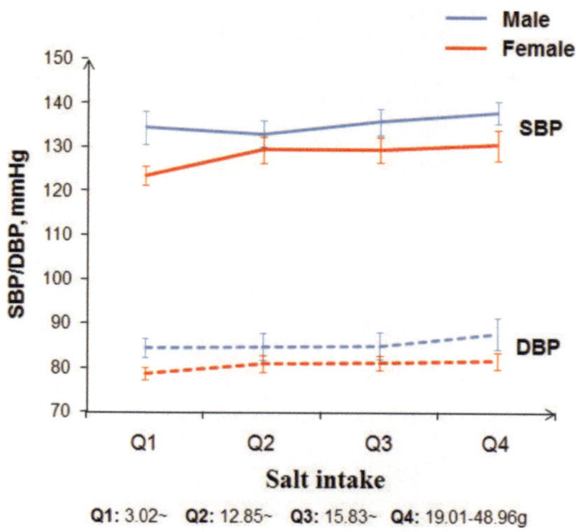

Figure 4. Estimated salt intake and BP in Kazakh people not taking antihypertensives (n = 1445).

high BP prevalence was also found when using a nonconditional logistic model (**Table 6**). A significantly increased prevalence for high BP was observed in the top quartile of urinary sodium excretion compared with the bottom quartile across the three different models. However, the strength of the association decreased after adjusting for potential confounding factors. In model 1 (adjusted for age only), ORs were 1.83 (95% CI: 1.19–2.83) and 2.38 (95% CI: 1.43–3.96) for men and women, respectively, in Q4 urinary sodium compared with Q1 (model 1). When the model was adjusted for residence, educational level, alcohol consumption, smoking, BMI, and fruit and vegetable consumption, the association between urinary sodium and prevalence for high BP attenuated, with ORs being 1.61 (95% CI: 1.02–2.54) for men and 1.92 (95% CI: 1.13–3.27) for women. Moreover, we found a much poor situation in people with controlled hypertension (2.9% for a BP control and 10.1% for a BP control under medication). There was an obviously increasing trend on treatment and control of hypertension following a sequence of nomads, farmers, and urban people, though this trend was not significant on control of hypertension (**Table 7**).

3.2. Occurrence of acute cardiovascular events

Forty-two cases with 46 acute cardiovascular events, including 7 acute myocardial infarctions, [14] 3 sudden cardiac deaths, and 36 incident strokes, were found. Among these events, there were four patients experiencing multiple acute cardiovascular events: one patient with two concurrent events, subarachnoid hemorrhage (SAH) and AMI; one patient with a nonfatal AMI and an in-hospital SCD after 31 days of the AMI occurrence; and two patients with ischemic stroke followed by another ischemic stroke or SAH after 28 days of the first stroke. All nonfatal AMIs had diagnostic evidence of markers of myocardial injury and ECG. 3 fatal cases were classified as possible AMIs with insufficient data. Besides one in-hospital SCD, 2 out-of -hospital SCDs were unwitnessed at the occurrence of death but observed alive within 24 hours from their death. All strokes, hemorrhagic or ischemic, had evidence of computed tomography (CT)

	Adjusted OR (95% CI) by gender	
	Men	**Women**
Model 1 adjusted for age		
Q1	1.00	1.00
Q2	1.05 (0.68,1.63)	1.58 (0.93,2.68)
Q3	1.06 (0.69,1.63)	1.66 (1.00,2.80)
Q4	1.83 (1.19,2.83)	2.38 (1.43,3.96)
Model 2 adjusted for age, occupation, and educational level		
Q1	1.00	1.00
Q2	1.05 (0.68,1.63)	1.38 (0.81,2.37)
Q3	1.95 (0.68,1.63)	1.45 (0.85,2.47)
Q4	1.81 (1.17,2.79)	2.06 (1.22,3.47)
Model 3 adjusted for age, occupation, educational level, body mass index, current smoker, current drinker, fruit consumption and vegetable consumption		
Q1	1.00	1.00
Q2	1.01 (0.64, 1.60)	1.29 (0.74, 2.23)
Q3	0.98 (0.62, 1.54)	1.30 (0.75, 2.24)
Q4	1.61 (1.02, 2.54)	1.92 (1.13, 3.27)

Table 6. Relationship between estimated salt intake and high BP (also see our previous publication [13]).

	Percent (95% CI)			
	Awareness	**Treatment**	**Controlled**	**Medication-controlled**
Nomad	60.7 (59.3–62.0)	24.8 (22.9–26.6)	2.2 (2.0–2.3)	8.8 (8.4–9.1)
Farmer	62.7 (61.5–63.9)	31.4 (29.4–33.3)	3.2 (3.1–3.4)	10.3 (9.9–10.6)
Urban people	52.5 (49.5–55.4)	34.4 (29.5–39.3)	4.9 (4.3–5.5)	14.3 (13.3–15.3)
P for trend	0.410	0.002	0.082	0.237
Total	61.0 (60.2–61.9)	28.8 (27.5–30.1)	2.9 (2.8–3.0)	10.1 (9.8–10.4)

Table 7. Awareness, treatment, and control of hypertension.

or magnetic resonance imaging (MRI). There were two cases with nonspecified stroke that was identified according to clinical manifestation. During this study, 31 deaths were found in 1668 individuals including 19 CVD underlying deaths (61.2%). Among 42 events, 17 deaths were followed in which 12, including 3 SCDs (I46.1), 2 SAHs (I60), 2 hemorrhagic strokes (I61), 2 acute cerebrovascular accidents (I64), and 3 coronary deaths with insufficient data, happened within 28 days after CVD occurrence.

In the electronic search for medical records in hospitals, repeated in-hospital records, particularly for nonacute ischemic stroke (I63), were common. One among the ischemic strokes listed in the second diagnosis, the first diagnosis being primary hypertension (stage 3), was identified as an acute event only. **Table 8** displays a comparison of the detailed search course for available files between the People's Hospital of Altay Prefecture and the People's Hospital of Altay City. Few AMIs shown in the People's Hospital of Altay City were in accordance with its ability for treating CVDs, dramatically different from most strokes likely due to a policy of referrals; this finding should be compared with the People's Hospital of Altay Prefecture, which ranks the highest in the Altay region. The number of events found in the People's Hospital of Altay Prefecture, the People's Hospital of Altay City, the 16th People's Liberation Army Hospital, and the Kazakh Hospital of Altay was 20, 7, 0, and 1, respectively; another 18 events (39.1%) were supplemented in the community. Among these 18 events, 5, 4, 1, 0, and 2 events were diagnosed in the four hospitals above and a tertiary hospital in Urumqi, Capital of Xinjiang, respectively, and 2, 1, and 3 events were classified as SCD, acute cerebrovascular accidents, and AMI with insufficient data, respectively. The proportion of fatal events supplemented by communities was significantly higher than that registered by hospitals (75.0% vs. 26.5%, $P = 0.003$). The ratio of events was 3.6:1 for stroke and cardiac events and this ratio was 1.6:1 for ischemic or hemorrhagic strokes. The detailed results are shown in **Table 9**.

A variation from the incidence of acute cardiovascular events following time and place is shown in **Table 10**. The incidence increased following time with a statistical significance ($P < 0.001$). As no events were identified in the township office and its adjacent Wutubulak village, we rechecked the information from the office by telephone through village physicians;

Search aim	The hospital of prefecture (Jan 2014–July 2016)		The hospital of city (Oct 2013–July 2016)	
	Records	Events	Records	Events
I21	1	0	0	0
I22	0	0	1	0
I46.1	0	0	0	0
I60	3	1	0	0
I61	10	4	4	0
I62	0	0	0	0
I63	13	5	114	5
I64	0	1	3	0
All-cause deaths	2	0	2	0

Table 8. Results of a search for medical records in 2 major hospitals, Altay.

CVD event	Hospital-based number (%)	Community-based number supplemented (%)	Total
Disease category			
Acute cardiac event			
Acute myocardiac infarction (I21~I22)	4 (57.1)	3 (42.9)	7
Sudden cardiac death (I46.1)	1 (33.3)	2 (66.6)	3
Subtotal	5 (50.0)	5 (50.0)	10
Acute stroke event			
SAH (I60)	1 (50.0)	1 (50.0)	2
Intracerebral hemorrhage (I61)	8 (62.7)	3 (27.3)	11
Other nontraumatic intracerebral hemorrhage (I62)	0	0	0
Cerebral infarction (I63)	13 (61.9)	8 (38.1)	21
Not specified as hemorrhage or infarction (I64)	1 (50.0)	1 (50.0)	2
Subtotal	23 (63.9)	13 (36.1)	36
Outcome category			
Non-fatal	25 (73.5)	9 (26.5)	34
Fatal	3 (25.0)	9 (75.0)	12
Total	28 (60.9)	18 (39.1)	46

Table 9. Comparison of hospital-based and community-based registration.

	Number of CVD events	Interval (years)	Number of all-cause deaths	Average population size	Crude incidence (per 10,0000)
Time of occurrence					
Oct 2012–Sep 2013	10	1.00	5	1665.5	600
Oct 2013–Sep 2014	13	1.00	7	1659.5	783
Oct 2014–Sep 2015	12	1.00	9	1651.5	727
Oct 2015–Jun 2016	11	0.75	10	1642.0	893
Village or township office					
Kesirjia	3	3.75	4	145.0	552
Tarstark	7	3.75	5	209.5	891
Bitiworg	14	3.75	8	274.0	1363
Wutubulak	9	3.75	4	191.0	1257
Sarkamus	10	3.75	7	373.5	714
Duolart	3	3.75	2	269.0	297
Township office	0	3.75	1	190.5	0
Total	46	3.75	31	1652.5	742

Table 10. Distribution of events by time and place.

http://dx.doi.org/10.5772/intechopen.69347

no new event was found. This could relate to a small population size, young age, and a low proportion of men. The incidence and mortality of acute cardiovascular events were highly affected by age. An incidence summit occurred in people aged 50–59 years (**Table 11**). In general, the crude rates of incidence and mortality for acute cardiovascular events were 742 and 194 per 100,000 people, respectively; the standardized rates were 926 and 272 per 100,000 people, respectively.

This part is also shown in our Chinese publication [15].

	Number by disease		Number by outcome		Total
	Cardiac event	Stroke	Nonfatal	Fatal	
Gender					
Male (%)	6 (60.0)	20 (55.6)	20 (58.8)	6 (50.0)	26 (56.5)
Female (%)	4 (40.0)	16 (44.4)	14 (41.2)	6 (50.0)	20 (43.5)
Incident age (years)					
< 40 (%)	1 (10.0)	2 (5.6)	2 (5.9)	1 (8.3)	3 (6.5)
40 ~ 49 (%)	1 (10.0)	7 (19.4)	6 (17.6)	2 (16.7)	8 (17.4)
50 ~ 59 (%)	3 (30.0)	11 (30.6)	10 (29.4)	4 (32.4)	14 (30.4)
60 ~ 69 (%)	2 (20.0)	7 (19.4)	8 (23.5)	1 (8.3)	9 (19.6)
70 ~ 79 (%)	0	9 (25.0)	8 (23.5)	1 (8.3)	9 (19.6)
≥ 80 (%)	3 (30.0)	0	0	3 (25.0)	3 (6.5)

Table 11. Distribution of events by gender and age.

4. Discussion

4.1. Epidemic of cardiovascular risk factors

The overall prevalence of cardiovascular risk factors was found to be high in this sample of Kazakh population, and varied markedly across occupational backgrounds. Compared with nomad and farmer groups, urban participants had more multiple cardiovascular risk factors and higher prevalence of dyslipidemia and obesity, while nomads possessed the highest prevalence of hypertension. The prevalence of diabetes mellitus was generally low in all subgroups which exhibited a separate status in these highly related indicators which normally coexist in cluster. Additionally, a higher prevalence of cardiovascular risk factors was associated with lower level annual family income and education attainment.

Previous studies on Kazakh populations considered Kazakh individuals as a single group, usually with comparisons to other ethnic groups [16–20]. Our study addressed a gap in intergroup variations in individual cardiovascular risk factor prevalence, which had several notable characteristics similar to previous work. First, Kazakh people were experiencing a strikingly higher rate of hypertension (50.1%); this prevalence is significantly higher than the national average (27.2% for a population aged 35 to 74 years) [18], higher than other ethnic groups such as Uygur (29.2%) and Han (30.2%) who account for 86% of total Xinjiang population, and also higher than previous reports for Kazakh adults (40.2%). Unfortunately, these people had a much poorer treatment and control of hypertension, compared with national average (28.8 vs. 82.9% for treatment of hypertension; 2.9 vs. 9.7% for BP control) [21]. In addition to differences in genetic backgrounds, dietary intake of high salt and high fat appeared to be major environmental factors that contributed to high BP in this ethnic group, especially for Kazakh nomads; this is supported by this study and our previous study [13]. Besides rare intake of vegetable and fruit, salty air-dried meat and milk-tea were their indispensable daily food and beverage. Estimated 24-h salt intake (20.6% of the person's salt intake came from drinking salty milk tea, a daily drink) with an average of 17.6 g/d was much higher than 12.4 g from WHO-CARDIAC study conducted in the same area (Kazakh as whole) in 2000 [22]. Salt-restriction, an easy, effective and affordable public health intervention, was needed urgently for these people. Second, urban participants had the highest prevalence of dyslipidemia compared with farmer and nomads groups, and this trend did not change following an increased age. Unlike some other studies showing that the prevalence of dyslipidemia in adult men changed with age like a "∩" shape [23–25], our results showed that young men possessed the highest prevalence of dyslipidemia and decreased significantly thereafter. For urban men, for example, the prevalence of dyslipidemia was 59.1% at age 30–44 years, 52.2% at age 45–59 years, and 33.3% at age ≥ 60 years. This trend may be explained by some social habits. In Kazakh, men rather than women had more chance to contact society, especially young men, they may be closely associated with men's social roles and have a higher chance to encounter unhealthy habits, including smoking, drinking (the prevalence of smoking and drinking was also at peak in this age period), and overeating as a result of social interaction, increasing the risk of dyslipidemia. With increasing age and reduced social interaction, awareness to protect one's health increases, leading to the reduction of dyslipidemia risk. For women, our results revealed a similar trend with other studies [23–25]. The prevalence of dyslipidemia in women initially decreased and subsequently increased, this trend might be closely related to changes in hormone levels [26]. Some studies indicated that sex hormone level was an independent risk factor for dyslipidemia [27]. Third, The overall prevalence of diabetes was generally low (1.56%) in this study, which was similar with previous Kazakh reports (1.47–3.65%) [28, 29], but much lower than 9.7% of the national average level [30]. Unlike previous studies, which reported that diabetes tended to be bundled with hypertension, and that there was substantial overlap between diabetes mellitus and hypertension in etiology and disease mechanisms, our results revealed that diabetes mellitus was a relatively independent disease, and 3.1% of hypertension patients had a coinstantaneous type 2 diabetes mellitus. The mechanism why Kazakh people have such low prevalence remains unclear; further study should be warranted.

Assessing the pattern of risk factors for CVDs in the Kazakh population is important for several reasons. First, despite rapid urbanization in China, most of Chinese people still live in rural areas, especially in ethnic minority communities. A Kazakh level of urbanization is 15.3%, which is much lower than the national average level (36.9%) [31]. Contrary to the prevailing belief among policy makers that cardiovascular risk factors primarily afflict the urban affluent, the burden of cardiovascular risk factors in rural areas of developing countries is currently heavy and rising [32], where people in resource-poor areas have less access to preventive services, less access to medication and procedures, and more exposure to risk factors. Understanding the distributions of cardiovascular risk factors in these populations is vital for planning public health responses. Second, China is a multiethnic country, with Tibetans and Mongolians, who live in Xinjiang, Tibet, Qinghai, and Inner Mongolia, which account for one-third of the total area of China; they have a lifestyle similar to that of Kazakh people. In addition to the possible effects of genetic background differences, environmental stress and lifestyle characteristics may have important effects on human physiology. These data provide important insights for the development of chronic diseases in populations who have similar living, environmental, and cultural exposures. Third, such data may contribute to our understanding of disease etiology by comparing risk profiles of naturally occurring groups. For example, persons with just one cardiovascular risk factor were more common in nomads or farmers, whereas those with ≥ 2 (for women ≥ 3) risk factors were more common in city people, which exhibits a clear way (from nomad to farmer to city people) showing that Kazakh people are experiencing lifestyle changes compared to the simple nomadic lifestyle and dietary habits; these changes are more conspicuous among young people. The genetic homogeneity of these groups tends to help isolate the role of environmental and lifestyle factors in the etiology of various chronic diseases.

4.2. Registration of acute cardiovascular events

Our preliminary work on registration of acute cardiovascular events has two main findings.

This work is highly complicated and needs coordination from public health and clinical specialists. Searching all probable incident clues and making a diagnosis for targeted cases are comparably important. To accumulate experience for a national surveillance of acute cardiovascular events that are not based on a cohort, we initially used a follow-up-based method by telephone. Hospital-based and community-based searches for CVD clues were synchronously employed, as suggested by the WHO MONICA project [33]. In this study, village physicians played an important role. They were familiar with health problems of local people and could provide some crude information on our interest after simple training. This reduced false negatives which might be caused due to seeing a doctor out of the local place, failing to search files in hospitals, and occurrence of death before arriving at hospital or at home. During a work stage in hospital, multiple files indexed by one patient code were boring; this was particularly frequent for ischemic stroke. Unfortunately, we could not directly access information on acute symptom, diagnostic evidence, and time of occurrence in a discharge card that usually is used by a hospital information system; this was serious in stroke that had a good match between ICD-10 code and a clinical diagnosis. With this situation, a disease history described in the medical records need to be read.

Studies related to incidence or mortality of acute cardiovascular events in Kazakh people are currently scarce. This population has a much higher incidence and mortality of acute cardiovascular events, compared with an average level in China. According to a national survey conducted in people aged 20 years or older across China in 2010, the incidence and mortality of stroke were 246.8 and 114.8 per 100,000 people standardized to China Census Population 2010, respectively [34]. The incidence of AMIs is unknown at the same time; however, related guidelines indicated that the ratio between AMIs and stroke was likely appropriate 1:5 [6] and this ratio was consistent with our study. Our study showed a 1.6 ratio of ischemic stroke compared to hemorrhagic stroke; this was much lower than the national level (approximately equal to 3) [34] that could be related to a much higher prevalence of hypertension in the Kazakh population. The age summit for acute cardiovascular events was 50–59 years in our sample population, younger than the mean age of people with prevalent stroke (66.4 years) in the national survey.

4.3. Strength, limitation, and its future

A key strength of this study is that we have a high-quality study design and practice with a high response rate which helps to ensure good internal validity and a reasonable approach to extrapolation of study results. However, a number of limitations should be kept in mind when assessing the evidence provided by our study. First, the participants in the urban group are relatively younger, and have a higher SES compared with other urban residents; therefore, the prevalence of cardiovascular risk factors may be underestimated. Second, because the study is community-based, the problem of clustering of risk factors within families could lead to some error in risk estimation, future research will be needed in this aspect. Nevertheless, our study population was from a town; this may lead to a limitation for generalizing our results, but this should not compromise the internal validity of our findings.

Due to a limited study year, we do not further calculate the incidence and mortality in different occupational populations. The next stage of follow-ups will be conducted. Nevertheless, we have established a population base with a follow-up system for cardiovascular outcomes and a good relationship with local governments. The Mother Program, aiming to reduce salt intake, is currently being conducted by local department of health and population. First, village physicians, women village leaders, and teachers in this town, who participate in an intervention for villagers, will be trained by seminars, textbooks, and multimedia. Second, all women will participate in multiple trainings about knowledge of hypertension and its prevention as well as how to reduce daily salt intake and improve diet. For a better effect, we will visit each family and help them achieve a goal of salt-restriction. Third, two-hour classes on hypertensive healthcare will be added per term in all schools of this town. We will have a rounded evaluation including all baseline contents every other year. During a further follow-up, we schedule the goal at the end of this study including lowering daily salt intake to 10 g, lowering blood pressure by 10/5 mmHg, and a significant reduction in incidence due to cardiovascular outcomes. Researchers, clinical physicians, and government officials are involved in this program team.

We believe that long-term effects of this lifestyle improvement will benefit not only male and female all-age Kazakh population but also next Kazakh generations. Also, our quality work will provide experience to combine medicine-based evidence with current nationwide policies, such as China National Herdsmen Settling Program covering two-thirds of land territory in China, for benefiting related ethnic minorities, such as Tibetan and Mongolian people.

5. Conclusions

In conclusion, findings from the CAKH study demonstrate the pervasive burden of cardiovascular risk factors and related acute cardiovascular events and an urgent need for controlling and preventing these risk factors in Kazakh population, especially BP in Kazakh nomads.

Acknowledgements

The governments of Altay City and Hong Dun Town supported this project. Village physicians and nurses from the Hong Dun Township Health Centre and Kazakh college students from Xinjiang Medical University participated in this survey. He P, Kang W, Jia L, Qin H, Yu H, Jumabieke N, and Jiangtai S provided administrative, technical, and material support. He P is currently conducting governmental issues on the Mother Program related to this study. We thank all interviewees, institutions, and individuals mentioned above.

Author details

Jingmei Jiang[1]*, Mingtao Zhang[2], Lei Hou[3], Wei Han[1], Yong Tang[2], Shaohua Liang[2] and Weizhi Wang[2]

*Address all correspondence to: jingmeijiang@ibms.pumc.edu.cn

1 Department of Epidemiology and Biostatistics, Institute of Basic Medical Sciences Chinese Academy of Medical Sciences/School of Basic Medicine Peking Union Medical College, Beijing, China

2 The People's Hospital of Altay Prefecture, Xinjiang, China

3 National Center for Chronic and Noncommunicable Disease Control and Prevention, Chinese Center for Disease Control and Prevention, Beijing, China

References

[1] Yusuf S, Hawken S, Ounpuu S, Dans T, Avezum A, Lanas F, McQueen M, Budaj A, Pais P, Varigos J, Lisheng L. Effect of potentially modifiable risk factors associated with myocardial infarction in 52 countries (the INTERHEART study): Case-control study. Lancet. 2004;**364**(9438):937-952. DOI: 10.1016/S0140-6736(04)17018-9

[2] O'Donnell MJ, Chin SL, Rangarajan S, Xavier D, Liu L, Zhang H, Rao-Melacini P, Zhang X, Pais P, Agapay S, Lopez-Jaramillo P, Damasceno A, Langhorne P, McQueen MJ, Rosengren A, Dehghan M, Hankey GJ, Dans AL, Elsayed A, Avezum A, Mondo C, Diener HC, Ryglewicz D, Czlonkowska A, Pogosova N, Weimar C, Iqbal R, Diaz R, Yusoff K, Yusufali A, Oguz A, Wang X, Penaherrera E, Lanas F, Ogah OS, Ogunniyi A, Iversen HK,

Malaga G, Rumboldt Z, Oveisgharan S, Al Hussain F, Magazi D, Nilanont Y, Ferguson J, Pare G, Yusuf S; INTERSTROKE Investigators. Global and regional effects of potentially modifiable risk factors associated with acute stroke in 32 countries (INTERSTROKE): A case-control study. Lancet. 2016;**388**(10046):761-775. DOI: 10.1016/S0140-6736(16)30506-2

[3] Hou L, Zhang M, Han W, Tang Y, Xue F, Liang S, Zhang B, Wang W, Asaiti K, Wang Y, Pang H, Wang Z, Wang Y, Qiu C, Jiang J. Influence of salt intake on association of blood uric acid with hypertension and related cardiovascular risk. PLoS One. 2016;**11**(4):e0150451. DOI: 10.1371/journal.pone.0150451

[4] Kawano Y, Tsuchihashi T, Matsuura H, Ando K, Fujita T, Ueshima H, Working Group for Dietary Salt Reduction of the Japanese Society of Hypertension. Report of the Working Group for Dietary Salt Reduction of the Japanese Society of Hypertension: (2) Assessment of salt intake in the management of hypertension. Hypertension Research. 2007;**30**(10):887-893

[5] The Chinese Work Group on Blood Pressure Measurements. Chinese guidelines on blood pressure measurements. Journal of Clinical Hypertension. 2011;**19**(12):1101-1114. Chinese

[6] Writing Group of 2010 Chinese Guidelines for the Management of Hypertension. 2010 Chinese guidelines for the management of hypertension. Journal of Clinical Hypertension. 2011;**19**(8):1101-1114. Chinese

[7] Joint Committee for Developing Chinese Guidelines on Prevention and Treatment of Dyslipidemia in Adults. Chinese guidelines on prevention and treatment of dyslipidemia in adults. Chinese Journal of Cardiology. 2007;**35**(5):390-419. Chinese

[8] Hou L, Han W, Jiang J, Liu B, Wu Y, Zou X, Xue F, Chen Y, Zhang B, Pang H, Wang Y, Wang Z, Hu Y, Li J. Passive smoking and stroke in men and women: A national population-based case-control study in China. Scientific Reports. 2017;**7**:45542. DOI: 10.1038/srep45542

[9] Wu Z, Yao C, Zhao D, Wu G, Wang W, Liu J, Zeng Z, Wu Y. Sino-MONICA project: A collaborative study on trends and determinants in cardiovascular diseases in China, Part I: Morbidity and mortality monitoring. Circulation. 2001;**103**(3):462-468

[10] Thygesen K, Alpert J, Jaffe A, Simoons M, Chaitman B, White H; Writing Group on Behalf of the Joint ESC/ACCF/AHA/WHF Task Force for the Universal Definition of Myocardial Infarction. Third universal definition of myocardial infarction. Circulation. 2012;**126**(8):2020-2025. DOI: 10.1161/CIR.0b013e31826e1058

[11] Chugh SS, Reinier K, Teodorescu C, Evanado A, Kehr E, Al Samara M, Mariani R, Gunson K, Jui J. Epidemiology of sudden cardiac death: Clinical and research implications. Progress Cardiovascular Disease. 2008;**51**(3):213-228. DOI: 10.1016/j.pcad.2008.06.003

[12] Jiang J, Zhang B, Zhang M, Xue F, Tang Y, Liang S, Hou L, Wang W, Han W, Asaiti K, Nasca PC, Wang Y, Pang H, Wang Z, Wang Y, Qiu C. Prevalence of conventional cardiovascular disease risk factors among Chinese Kazakh individuals of diverse occupational

backgrounds in Xinjiang China. International Journal of Cardiology. 2015;**179**:558-560. DOI: 10.1016/j.ijcard.2014.10.077

[13] Han W, Hu Y, Tang Y, Xue F, Hou L, Liang S, Zhang B, Wang W, Asaiti K, Pang H, Wang Z, Wang Y, Zhang M, Jiang J. Relationship between urinary sodium with blood pressure and hypertension among a Kazakh community population in Xinjiang, China. Journal of Human Hypertension. 2017;**31**(5):333-340. DOI: 10.1038/jhh.2016.83

[14] Thygesen K, Alpert JS, Jaffe AS, Simoons ML, Chaitman BR, White HD; Joint ESC/ACCF/AHA/WHF Task Force for the Universal Definition of Myocardial Infarction, Katus HA, Lindahl B, Morrow DA, Clemmensen PM, Johanson P, Hod H, Underwood R, Bax JJ, Bonow RO, Pinto F, Gibbons RJ, Fox KA, Atar D, Newby LK, Galvani M, Hamm CW, Uretsky BF, Steg PG, Wijns W, Bassand JP, Menasché P, Ravkilde J, Ohman EM, Antman EM, Wallentin LC, Armstrong PW, Simoons ML, Januzzi JL, Nieminen MS, Gheorghiade M, Filippatos G, Luepker RV, Fortmann SP, Rosamond WD, Levy D, Wood D, Smith SC, Hu D, Lopez-Sendon JL, Robertson RM, Weaver D, Tendera M, Bove AA, Parkhomenko AN, Vasilieva EJ, Mendis S. Third universal definition of myocardial infarction. Circulation. 2012;**126**(16):2020-2035. DOI: 10.1161/CIR.0b013e31826e1058

[15] Hou L, Han W, Tang Y, Xue F, Liang S, Wang W, Zhang B, Pang H, Wang Y, Wang Z, Hu Y, Wang L, Zhang M, Jiang J. A pilot study to explore a registry method for acute cardiovascular events. National Medicine Journal of China. 2017;**97**(13):1024-1029. Chinese

[16] Wu Y, Huxley R, Li L, Anna V, Xie G, Yao C, Woodward M, Li X, Chalmers J, Gao R, Kong L, Yang X, China NNHS Steering Committee; China NNHS Working Group. Prevalence, awareness, treatment, and control of hypertension in China: Data from the China National Nutrition and Health Survey 2002. Circulation. 2008;**118**(25):2679-2686. DOI: 10.1161/CIRCULATIONAHA.108.788166

[17] Gu D, Reynolds K, Wu X, Chen J, Duan X, Muntner P, Huang G, Reynolds RF, Su S, Whelton PK, He J; InterASIA Collaborative Group. The International Collaborative Study of Cardiovascular Disease in ASIA. Prevalence, awareness, treatment, and control of hypertension in China. Hypertension. 2002;**40**(6):920-927

[18] Ma X, Zhang M, Guo S, Ma R, Ding Y, Guo H, Zhang J, Niu Q, Li S, Liu J, Xu S. Prevalence of hypertension in Uygur, Kazakhs and Han people in rural areas of Xinjiang. Chinese Journal of Hypertensions. 2013;**21**(12):1164-1168. Chinese

[19] Zhai F, He Y, Wang Z, Hu Y. Status and characteristic of dietary intake of 12 minority nationalities in China. Wei Sheng Yan Jiu. 2007;**36**(5):539-541. Chinese

[20] Li J, Wang L, Li Y, Bi Y, Jiang Y, Mi S, Dai M, Xu Y, Ning G, Zhao W. Epidemiologic characteristics of dyslipidemia in Chinese adults 2010. Zhonghua Yu Fang Yi Xue Za Zhi. 2012;**46**(5):414-418. Chinese

[21] Li Y, Yang L, Wang L, Zhang M, Huang Z, Deng Q, Zhou M, Chen Z, Wang L. Burden of hypertension in China: A nationally representative survey of 174,621 adults. International Journal of Cardiology. 2017;**227**:516-523. DOI: 10.1016/j.ijcard.2016.10.110

[22] Liu L, Liu L, Ding Y, Huang Z, He B, Sun S, Zhao G, Zhang H, Miki T, Mizushima S, Ikeda K, Nara Y, Yamori Y. Ethnic and environmental differences in various markers of dietary intake and blood pressure among Chinese Han and three other minority peoples of China: Results from the WHO Cardiovascular Diseases and Alimentary Comparison (CARDIAC) study. Hypertension Research. 2001;**24**(3):315-322

[23] Guo SX, Ma RL, Guo H, Ding YS, Liu JM, Zhang M, Zhang JY, Xu SZ, Li SG, Rui DS, Niu Q, Li YP. Epidemiological analysis of dyslipidemia in adults of three ethnicities in Xinjiang, China. Genetics and Molecular Research. 2014;**13**(2):2385-2393. DOI: 10.4238/2014.April.3.11

[24] Joshi SR, Anjana RM, Deepa M, Pradeepa R, Bhansali A, Dhandania VK, Joshi PP, Unnikrishnan R, Nirmal E, Subashini R, Madhu SV, Rao PV, Das AK, Kaur T, Shukla DK, Mohan V; ICMR-INDIAB Collaborative Study Group. Prevalence of dyslipidemia in urban and rural India: The ICMR-INDIAB study. PLoS One. 2014;**9**(5):e96808. DOI: 10.1371/journal.pone.0096808

[25] Cabrera M, Sánchez-Chaparro MA, Valdivielso P, Quevedo-Aguado L, Catalina-Romero C, Fernández-Labandera C, Ruiz-Moraga M, González-Santos P, Calvo-Bonacho E; ICARIA (Ibermutuamur CArdiovascular RIsk Assessment) Study Group. Prevalence of atherogenic dyslipidemia: Association with risk factors and cardiovascular risk in Spanish working population. "ICARIA" study. Atherosclerosis. 2014;**235**(2):562-569. DOI: 10.1016/j.atherosclerosis.2014.05.960

[26] Sowers MR, Randolph J Jr, Jannausch M, Lasley B, Jackson E, McConnell D. Levels of sex steroid and cardiovascular disease measures in premenopausal and hormone-treated women at midlife: Implications for the "timing hypothesis". Archives of Internal Medicine. 2008;**168**(19):2146-2153. DOI: 10.1001/archinte.168.19.2146

[27] Ali ZA, Al-Zaidi MS. The association between body mass index, lipid profile and serum estradiol levels in a sample of Iraqi diabetic premenopausal women. Oman Medical Journal. 2011;**26**(4):263-266

[28] Yang YN, Xie X, Ma YT, Li XM, Fu ZY, Ma X, Huang D, Chen BD, Liu F, Huang Y, Liu C, Zheng YY, Baituola G, Yu ZX, Chen Y. Type 2 diabetes in Xinjiang Uygur autonomous region, China. PLoS One. 2012;**7**(4):e35270. DOI: 10.1371/journal.pone.0035270

[29] Tao Y, Mao X, Xie Z, Ran X, Liu X, Wang Y, Luo X, Hu M, Gen W, Zhang M, Wang T, Ren J, Wufuer H, Li L. The prevalence of type 2 diabetes and hypertension in Uygur and Kazak populations. Cardiovascular Toxicology. 2008;**8**(4):155-159. DOI: 10.1007/s12012-008-9024-0

[30] Yang W, Lu J, Weng J, Jia W, Ji L, Xiao J, Shan Z, Liu J, Tian H, Ji Q, Zhu D, Ge J, Lin L, Chen L, Guo X, Zhao Z, Li Q, Zhou Z, Shan G, He J; China National Diabetes and Metabolic Disorders Study Group. Prevalence of diabetes among men and women in China. The New England Journal of Medicine. 2010;**362**(12):1090-1101. DOI: 10.1056/NEJMoa0908292

[31] National Bureau of Statistics of China. The data of the fifth population census in China. 2000. Available from: Http://www.stats.gov.cn/tjsj/ndsj/renkoupucha/2000pucha/pucha.htm

[32] Myers L, Mendis S. Cardiovascular disease research output in WHO priority areas between 2002 and 2011. Journal of Epidemiology and Global Health. 2014;**4**(1):23-28

[33] Tunstall-Pedoe H. Problems with criteria and quality control in the registration of coronary events in the MONICA study. Acta Medica Scandinavica. 1988;**728**(Suppl.):17-25

[34] Wang W, Jiang B, Sun H, Ru X, Sun D, Wang L, Wang L, Jiang Y, Li Y, Wang Y, Chen Z, Wu S, Zhang Y, Wang D, Wang Y, Feigin VL; NESS-China Investigators. Prevalence, incidence and mortality of stroke in China: Results from a nationwide population-based survey of 480,687 adults. Circulation. 2017. DOI: 10.1161/CIRCULATIONAHA.116.025250

Chapter 3

Overview of Some Risk Factors in Cardiovascular Disease

Elena Cojocaru, Alexandra Mastaleru,
Bogdan Tamba, Raluca Vasile,
Razvan Cosmin Tudor, Carmen Valerica Ripa,
Roxana Cobzaru and Maria Magdalena Leon

Additional information is available at the end of the chapter

http://dx.doi.org/10.5772/intechopen.69039

Abstract

Much more specialists are nowadays aligning themselves on the view according to which the prevalence of cardiovascular disease will reach epidemic levels in the near future due to the increase of hypertension, diabetes and obesity. Most epidemiological studies indicate that we are confronted with a multiplication of risk factors, with an emphasis on their genetic conditioning as well as an acceleration of the effects generated by non-genetic factors. According to WHO recommendations, the appropriate methods of reducing the cardiovascular risk are those that combine health policies with efficient education measures. Long-term results of these measures aim to decrease the incidence of complications and associated costs with their treatment at the same time with increasing the quality of life. Approximately 50% of deaths from heart disease could be prevented through sustained action on the main cause—hypertension—and by treating risk factors, primarily hyperlipidemia and elevated body weight. Atherosclerotic disease requires a rigorous approach because identifying predisposing risk factors with proven implications in the initiation and progression of this disease, as well as modulation of those with protective role, can have a significant impact in finding an appropriate treatment in order to improve cardiovascular diseases and their consequences.

Keywords: hypertension, diabetes, obesity, atherosclerosis, metabolic syndrome

1. Introduction

Significant research has suggested that vascular segments that have fingerprints of the atherosclerotic lesions (endothelial dysfunctions, macrophage activation, cellular proliferation and thrombosis) respond differently on medication, starting from the idea that we can accept as a initial point either inflammation or normal lipid profile perturbation [1, 2]. Therapeutic approach of the atherogenic dyslipidemia imposes the correlation with proatherogenic individual tendencies in order to correct the further risks. Atherosclerosis must be seen as a continuous process that starts from small endothelial dysfunctions and leads to important alterations of the vascular wall [3, 4]. The use of pharmacotherapeutic agents must be done in a tight correlation with the local pathophysiology, evaluating not only the risk factors but also the dynamic knowledge and clinical manifestations of this global disease [5, 6]. Although there are certain atherogenic risk factors considered causal agents for atherosclerosis, this disease can appear and evolve in their absence. Thus, there have been revealed atherosclerotic plaques in patients deceased from ischemic cardiomyopathy and especially from myocardial infarction, regardless of the blood pressure values, or the cholesterol and triglycerides values, and the presence or absence of smoking [7].

2. Main body

Myocardial infarction, stroke and venous thromboembolism represent the most important causes of death among female and men. Coronary heart disease, due to atherosclerosis, is a cause of myocardial infarction and is the first cause of death in women and men worldwide [7]. Strokes by venous or arterial thrombosis are more frequently in menopausal woman, whereas the stroke with cerebral hemorrhage, even if is less frequent, appears in young female and is caused by a cerebral vascular anomaly. Venous thrombosis includes superficial thrombosis that are autolimitated and deep thrombosis, most frequently at the level of popliteal and femoral vein. In approximately 10% of cases, a part of the thrombus or the entire thrombus can detach and determine pulmonary embolism [8].

Cardiovascular disease appears in coronary arteries when the atherosclerotic lesions evolve from an initial accumulation of isolated foam cells in the arterial intima to fatty streaks, followed by the accumulation of cholesterol deposits and atheroma formation. Once the atheroma is formed, the collagen from the fibrous cap stabilizes the plaque and prevents its rupture. But, matrix metalloproteinases, which are produced by the inflammatory cells from the lesion level, may degrade the collagen, and in case of a rupture of the fibrous cap, the resulted thrombus can block the affected coronary artery [9].

Cardiovascular disease may have their origin in the intrauterine life, but also a low birth weight and an extremely rich diet increase the risk of obesity and a specific metabolic syndrome in adults. Cardiovascular disease incidence and mortality are very low in reproductive age women, but it increases with age [8].

Estradiol (E2) reduces the development of the early atherosclerotic lesions, in some measure, by its effects on the lipid metabolism, with a reduction of the lipid deposits from the intima. On the other hand, at the level of the already made atheroma, the estrogens increase the matrix metalloproteinases expression, which can lead to the disruption of the fibrous cap and the rupture of the plaque. In this case, a turbulent blood flow is produced; the estradiol has thrombogenic properties and leads to clot formation that may obstruct the arterial lumen [10]. Therefore, through various mechanisms, the estrogens inhibit the early development of the atherosclerosis but at the same time increase the risk of complications once the atherosclerosis has been installed. Atherosclerotic lesions from the carotids and cerebral vessels may be affected by similar mechanisms; thus, in comparison with men, women are relatively protected by the thrombotic stroke before menopause, and any hormonal impact leads to changes in the status of the coagulation, anticoagulation and thrombotic factors [11].

World Health Organization conducted numerous studies regarding the mortality due to myocardial infarction, stroke and venous thromboembolism in many countries across the world [12]. Mortality by myocardial infarction in women increases exponentially with age. It is twice as high in American population as in the West Pacific population. The mortality rate of this condition is smaller in reproductive aged people, being 1–7 in 100,000 women aged 35–44 years/year. Reproductive aged women have 3–5 times smaller mortality rates than men, becoming similar over the age of 65 years. Consequently, age has a major influence because the number and the severity of the lesions increase with age; for this reason, the prevention of the atherosclerosis progression is very important, even in the seventh or eighth decade of life [13]. Atherosclerosis is not symptomatic until midlife or later, when the arterial lesions determine organ injury. However, cardiovascular signaling markers were frequently identified in children in the last few years. Anatomopathological examination of coronary arteries sampled from children who died in accidents showed fatty streaks and fibrous caps, in smoking, high blood pressure, obese or dyslipidemic subjects. Therefore, it is mandatory to identify the risk factors at an early age in order to prevent the premature appearance of myocardial infarction [14, 15]. Epidemiological studies revealed an increased incidence of myocardial infarction approximately five times higher in individuals between the ages of 40 and 60 years [16].

Hormonal contraceptives, pregnancy and polycystic ovary syndrome in young women and menopause in older women are directly linked with cardiovascular diseases [17]. The use of combined hormonal contraceptives has minor effects in cardiovascular disease, given the low incidence of myocardial infarction, stroke and venous thromboembolism in young women. However, women who already have risk factors or cardiovascular diseases should take into consideration alternative contraceptive methods. In pregnant women, cardiovascular diseases are rare; even in West countries they determine a significant proportion of maternal mortality compared to the substantial decrease of obstetrical mortality. The frequency of venous thromboembolism is 15 in 10,000 in pregnancy and post-partum period [18]. In older woman, it seems that menopause determines a higher risk of myocardial infarction, even if the results of numerous studies show a significant risk of heterogeneity. It is known that estrogen reduces the risk of developing atherosclerosis in premenopausal women, whereas in post-menopause, in women with atherosclerotic disease, the estrogen increases the risk of myocardial disease by its effects over the plaque stability and clot forming. The recent study results indicate that hormonal treatment in menopause does not always improve the risk of myocardial infarction, stroke or other vascular diseases. Thus, cardiovascular disease prevention should be based on diet and sport, small doses of platelet antiaggregant and treatment of high blood pressure, hyperglycemia and hyperlipidemia [19, 20].

The atherosclerosis complications are unusual in premenopausal women, with the exception of the ones predisposed to diabetes mellitus, hyperlipidemia or high blood pressure. The incidence of diseases related to atherosclerosis increases in menopause, probably being connected to the disappearance of the hormonal protection [16]. Some data demonstrated that estrogen replacement therapy has a favorable effect over the risk, increasing HDL and decreasing LDL levels [21]. The use of steroid hormonal contraceptives increases two to three times coronary atherosclerosis risk, mainly in smoking female over 35 years [22].

In the last few years, the criteria for metabolic syndrome have been reviewed: abdominal obesity, increased serum cholesterol, high blood pressure, insulin resistance with or without impaired glucose tolerance, pro-inflammatory status, a high level of C-reactive protein and a prothrombotic status with a high plasmatic fibrinogen and coagulation factors level [23].

Morphological and experimental studies have demonstrated connections between hyperlipidemia, especially hypercholesterolemia, and atherosclerosis, both in women and in men. The content of the atheroma plaque, which is made of cholesterol and cholesterol esters, the structure of the foam cells and the experimental production of atherosclerosis by a high-fat diet, has been initial arguments for the implication of lipids in atherosclerosis genesis. Cholesterol and triglycerides are the lipids with the highest impact for atherosclerosis and ischemic cardiomyopathy. Prospective studies showed that patients with a plasmatic cholesterol level over 260 mg% have a three or four times higher incidence of atherosclerosis than the patients with a level under 200 mg% [24]. From the total cholesterol, the major component that is associated with a high risk is LDL-cholesterol that has an essential physiological role in supplying the cholesterol to the peripheral tissue [25]. In opposition, HDL-cholesterol has the role of uptaking the cholesterol from the forming atheroma or from those already formed and transport it to the liver. Beside the ability of removing the cholesterol from the cellular level, HDL-cholesterol has anti-inflammatory, antioxidant and antithrombotic properties that contribute to the improvement of the endothelial function and atherosclerosis inhibition. Therefore, as the HDL-cholesterol level is higher, the risk of developing atherosclerosis lowers [26, 27]. In different experimental models, carbohydrate restriction proved to be efficient in the decrease of the plasmatic triglycerides, increase of HDL-cholesterol and modifying the repartition of the LDL-cholesterol [28]. The physical exercises and moderate consume of ethanol increase the HDL-cholesterol level, whereas the obesity and smoking decrease it. High cholesterol diets or saturated fats, like the ones from the butter, animal fats and yolk, increase the level of the plasmatic cholesterol, whereas the diets poor in cholesterol and polyunsaturated fats decrease it. Omega-3 fatty acids, found in fish oil, are probably beneficial, whereas the unsaturated fats produced by the artificial hydrogenation of the vegetable polyunsaturated fats and used in alimentation may influence negatively the cholesterol profiles, conducting to atherosclerosis. Beneficial effects of the omega fatty acids have been observed in the Northern countries, where the consumption of a large quantity of fish determined a decrease of the cardiovascular disease. If the cholesterol value cannot be diminished by diet, we can use drugs named statins that reduce the indirect circulating cholesterol by inhibiting the HMGCoA-reductase, a key enzyme necessary for the biosynthesis of the cholesterol in the liver [16, 29, 30]. From the existing statins on the market, studies showed the efficacy in cardiovascular disease prevention for Atorvastatin and Rosuvastatin [31].

Early coronary artery disease appears usually in patients with medical history of hypercholesterolemia. Numerous laboratory tests showed significantly higher levels of cholesterol and lower levels of HDL-cholesterol (especially of HDL2) in patients under 40 years old with coronary artery disease (men or women) compared to patients over 60 years old to whom the disease could be noticed [32].

The screening involves dosing cholesterol and LDL-cholesterol levels, and it is recommended to all the adults, especially to young people with a familial history of early ischemic cardiomyopathy. The actual dyslipidemia guideline highlights the importance of maintaining the LDL-cholesterol value within normal limits and reporting the cardiovascular disease to this value [33].

Polycystic ovary syndrome should be seen as a metabolic disease, with a high risk in developing diabetes mellitus type 2 and different cardiovascular disease [34]. If the glucose value is between 110 and 120 mg/dl, it is mandatory to perform the oral glucose tolerance test that allows us to precocious discover the diabetes mellitus and remove the complications. According to an international consent about the diagnostic criteria (The Rotterdam ESHRE/ASRM-Sponsored PCOS Consensus Workshop Group, 2004), this syndrome is characterized by oligomenorrhea/amenorrhea, hyperandrogenism and polycystic ovaries. In addition, this syndrome is frequently associated with obesity and insulin resistance. Although women with this syndrome require medical assistance for unregulated menstrual cycles, hirsutism and infertility, it should not neglect the high risk of developing cardiovascular disease; therefore, clinician attention should be directed also to long-term prevention over these diseases [35].

Recent clinical studies regarding this syndrome established the existence of some metabolic risk factors in these women. The intermediary results include endothelial dysfunction, platelet dysfunction, increased number of leukocytes or high levels of C-reactive protein, coronary calcifications and the increase of the intima-media thickness at the carotid level. A study conducted on 161 patients with polycystic ovary syndrome also established frequent alterations in the metabolic syndrome parameters [36]. Regarding intermediate results, 33 women aged between 40 and 59 years, with histological confirmed syndrome, have been followed up to 2–3 decades concluding that they developed obesity, high prevalence of diabetes mellitus and high blood pressure, compared with a same aged group [37].

Concerning the cardiovascular events, limited studies on females with polycystic ovary syndrome provided contradictory results, even if it has been established a certain correlation with a metabolic syndrome. We must highlight the fact that most studies are retrospective, on a small number of patients, on a short follow-up and a lot of questions regarding the control groups [38, 39]. Large prospective cohort studies, like Framingham or Nurses Health Study, focused over results about cardiovascular disease or cancers, could not identify hyperandrogenism and anovulation as a separate risk phenotype. If we talk about American population, they can calculate their death risk by cardiovascular disease using Framingham score. In Europe, we should take into consideration SCORE risk charts (Systematic Coronary Risk Evaluation Project). This allows each person to simply calculate his death risk by cardiovascular disease in the next 10 years. It has the advantage that is very easy to use and all we need to know is gender, age, smoking status, blood pressure and cholesterol level. It can be used by anybody and brings precious individualized information based on which it can be prescribed a treatment. A retrospective study from Great Britain, which included 786 women diagnosed with polycystic ovary syndrome between 1930 and 1979, could not establish the increase of the cardiovascular disease [40] or the morbidity [41] in these patients.

Cardiovascular disease is less frequent in women in reproductive age. First report regarding the cardiovascular disease as a secondary effect of the contraception took place in 1961, short after the discovery of the combined oral contraceptives [42]. Starting from 1960, estrogen and progesterone doses from contraceptive pills have been dramatically reduced and were created new progestatives that are theoretically safer. Substantial data regarding the effects of the combined oral contraceptives over the cardiovascular disease exist, but there are less evidence for the contraceptive pills that contain only progesterone [43].

High blood pressure is a condition characterized by an increase of the systolic value over 140 mmHg and of the diastolic value over 90 mmHg, being a major risk factor for atherosclerosis at all ages, females being less affected [16]. Prothrombotic condition and Lp(a) are two risk factors correlated with the development and the progression of the organic damage in high blood pressure and also in the evolution of the atherosclerotic process [44]. Antihypertensive drugs reduce the incidence of atherosclerosis-associated diseases, such as strokes and ischemic heart disease [45]. High blood pressure is a risk factor common in old people compared to young people with a myocardial infarction, frequently found in females [46]. Mechanisms by which the high blood pressure accelerates the atherogenesis include: the direct lesion of the endothelial cells from the susceptible zones from the mechanic stress exercised over the vascular lumen, the alteration of the endothelial permeability with the increase of the lysosomal enzymes activity, the gradual thickening of the arterial intima caused by the proliferation of the smooth muscle fiber and connective tissue components [16].

Another extremely important risk factor involved in women atherosclerosis is heredity. Variable damage of the genes together with the environmental factors determines a different atherogenic predisposition among the population. It has not been identified yet a genetic marker for atherosclerosis, but it seems that the genetic predisposed subjects for this degenerative disease are more vulnerable if associated with risk factors. Familial predisposition to atherosclerosis and ischemic heart disease is most probably polygenic [16] and normally is associated with other risk factors, like high blood pressure and diabetes mellitus. Familial risk for ischemic cardiomyopathy is extremely high in some dyslipidemia: familial hypercholesterolemia, polygenic hypercholesterolemia and polygenic hypoalphalipoproteinemia [47].

Numerous proatherogenic factors have been discovered in various studies. Apolipoprotein E, with its three principal variants (E2, E3, E4), is a good example of genetic polymorphism involved in the atherosclerotic process [48]. In different populations, it was demonstrated that Apo E polymorphism is a major determinant for coronary disease. The risk of myocardial infarction is smaller in patients with epsilon 2–E2 allele than the patients with epsilon 4–E4 allele [49]. A decreased frequency of epsilon 4 allele has been found in the Northern countries of Europe, whereas this increases in the Southern Europe, like the cardiovascular disease mortality rate. In addition, a strong relationship between the medical history and the epsilon 4 Apo E distribution was established. Despite normal LDL, HDL and total cholesterol values, Apo E polymorphism has been associated with negative prognostic, which raised the hypothesis that epsilon 4 allele represents a determinant factor for accelerated atherosclerosis in young people with myocardial infarction, by the modulation of other risk factors [50].

Decreased arterial compliance has a high predictive value for cardiovascular events, so its evaluation becomes an important objective in investigating the arterial function [51]. Various epidemiological and clinical studies brought arguments for a genetic component that is involved in the modulation of the arterial wall properties, unrelated with other risk factors [52]. An important number of genes that might affect the structure and role of the arterial wall exist (genes implied in different signaling paths and in modulating the extracellular matrix), and their identification is extremely important, offering on the one hand new biomarkers that are useful in evaluating the arterial compliance, and on the other hand new therapeutic targets in order to decrease the vascular rigidity [53, 54]. Currently, the arteriography allows the noninvasive quantification of vascular rigidity and long-term monitoring in cardiovascular rehabilitation programs.

Recent studies have shown that smoking is the most important adjustable risk factor in women and men under 40 years old with acute coronary syndrome, being observed in mostly equal parts in those with normal coronary arteries and in those with lesions on one or more coronary arteries [55]. Smoking is involved in endothelial dysfunction by reducing the production of the nitric oxide, causing the coronary spasm [37]. Smoking one pack a day or more than one pack for years increases the ischemic cardiac disease mortality rate up to 200%. Smoking cessation considerably reduces the risk of developing the disease [16, 56].

Diabetes mellitus induces hypercholesterolemia and in consequence an increase in predisposition for atherosclerosis in both male and female. The incidence of the myocardial infarction is two times higher at patients with diabetes mellitus compared to patients without diabetes. Also they have a higher risk for strokes and it increases almost 100 times the risk of the gangrene on the inferior limb, induced by atherosclerosis, being most often discovered at smoker patients with diabetes [16]. This disease affects the elastic properties of the arterial wall, no matter the presence of other risk factors or intimal damage in patients with peripheral vascular disease [57]. Acute hypoglycemia causes important physiological changes, affecting cardiovascular system and some hematological parameters, mainly as a consequence of the sympatho-adrenergic activation. In healthy adults, cardiovascular effects are transitory and do not have severe consequences, but can become pathological in patients with diabetes that already have endothelial dysfunction. The risk of localized tissue ischemia may be increased by acute hemodynamic and hematologic alterations; also, major vascular events like myocardial or cerebral ischemia may be precipitated by acute hypoglycemia [58]. Clinical and experimental studies sustain the idea that insulin resistance syndrome and increased levels of circulating insulin are involved in cardiac ischemic disease [59].

High blood pressure and diabetes mellitus are risk factors associated most of the time in patients with cardiovascular diseases. Impaired glucose tolerance is accompanied by an increase in the thickness and the rigidity of great vessels, which determines high blood pressure, macrovascular complications and decreased renal function [60]. Chronic hypertension and diabetes produce physiopathological changes both in great vessels and in microvascularization.

The increase of the arterial rigidity leads to increased systolic pressure and pulse pressure that conducts to a fall in the coronary perfusion. The remodeling of the resistance arteries and the capillary rarefaction causes the growth of the peripheral resistance, with high blood pressure and the amplification of the negative hemodynamic effects of the reduced arterial compliance; therefore, therapeutic interventions that must stop these vascular changes should have the aim to increase the central systolic pressure and the increase of the vascular bed perfusion [61, 62].

Patients with homocystinuria, which is a congenital metabolic disorder, characterized by elevated levels of circulating homocysteine (> 100 μmol/L) and urinary homocysteine, presents an early vascular injury [63]. Clinical and epidemiological studies revealed a connection between the serum levels of homocysteine and peripheral vascular disease, coronary artery disease, stroke, venous thrombosis, meaning that a high concentration of homocysteine is associated with the progression of the atherosclerosis [64]. Also, high concentrations of homocysteine imperil the endothelial function, increase the oxidative stress, affect the methylation reactions and alter the protein structures [63]. Hyperhomocysteinemia can be caused by the reduced absorption of the folic acid and B type vitamins and, in consequence, recent data suggest that folic acid and B6 vitamin ingestion, together with a proper diet, could reduce the incidence of cardiovascular disease, but this remains to be established in further studies [16]. An increase of homocysteine concentration is correlated with a 10% risk of coronary disease. The increase of homocysteine up to 5 micromol/L carries a 41% higher risk, similar to a cholesterol increase with 0.52 micromol/L (20 mg/L). Smoking and high blood pressure amplify the atherogenic action of high homocysteine levels. The association between hyperhomocysteine and factor V Leiden increases three to six times the thrombosis risk [65, 66].

A particular interest is conferred to the infectious etiology of atherosclerosis. Viral infections (herpes viruses, HIV-1), *Mycoplasma* or *Chlamydia* can affect the endothelial cell function and thus an increased adherence of the leukocytes and thrombocytes at the injured vascular section [67, 68]. Numerous studies showed that atherosclerosis can be the consequence of the adaptive immunity due to microbial HSP-60 (Heat Shock Protein-60). Stress factors induce the growth of the HSP expression on the endothelial cells and the cross-reactivity between the antibodies and the microbial HSP that lead to autoimmune reaction and accelerated atherosclerosis. The association between the infectious syndrome and coronary disease has been reported in many studies [69].

It has been issued the hypothesis that the infection of the vascular wall with pathogen agents like *Chlamydia pneumoniae* or cytomegalovirus (CMV) contributes to the appearance of atherosclerosis by insertion of new antigens in the vessel wall [70, 71]. *C. pneumoniae* was evidenced by direct immunofluorescence on endarterectomy pieces or by antibodies anti-*C. pneumoniae* in plasma. *Chlamydia pneumonia* and CMV were absent in non-atherosclerotic vessels. The use of antibiotics in certain infections limits the atherosclerotic process [72].

At vascular wall level where atherosclerosis appears, there is a particular accumulation of mononuclear cells, CD4+ and CD8+ lymphocytes [73]. Endothelial cells, macrophages and dendritic cells have a role of antigen-presenting cells [72]. Infectious agents can infect macrophages and persist for a long time at their level, producing proinflammatory cytokine (INF-γ,

TNF-α, IL-1, IL-6, IL-8), metalloproteinase and integrins [74, 75]. It is important to mention the antigenic mimetism between oxidized LDL and *Streptococcus pneumoniae*; subsequently, the vaccination with pneumococcal antigen induces an immune response against oxidized LDL that might immunomodulate the atherosclerosis process [76].

Other factors that are hard to evaluate include the physical effort, type A of personality (characterized by a stressed lifestyle), obesity; they determine high blood pressure, diabetes mellitus, hypertriglyceridemia and increase of LDL-cholesterol [16]. Regularly physical activity induces the increase of HDL-cholesterol, slowing the atherogenesis process and preventing ischemic cardiomyopathy. Physical and emotional stress and anxiety seem to be precipitating factors for ischemic heart disease and sudden death [77]. In Framingham study, cardiovascular disease incidence was two times higher in obese men and 2.5 times in obese women under 50 years old [78]. Adipose tissue considered for a long time just a fat source, seems to be a proinflammatory endocrine and paracrine secretion organ. It is recognized as being an important source of proinflammatory mediators that can contribute in vascular injury, insulin resistance and atherogenesis. So the inflammation of the adipose tissue can be an important step in developing numerous manifestations in connection with pathological characteristics of metabolic syndrome and may lead to diabetes and atherosclerosis [79, 80]. Defining a relevant obesity phenotype for cardiovascular risk can be done by adipocytokine identification, biomarkers that quantify the metabolic activity of the adipose tissue [81]. According to their effect, adipocytokines can be classified into proinflammatory adipocytokines, mediators of endothelial dysfunction and atherosclerosis that include TNF-α (tumor necrosis factor), IL-6 (interleukin 6), leptin, plasminogen activator inhibitor (PAI-1), angiotensinogen, resistin and C-reactive protein (CRP), and adipocytokines with antiatherosclerotic role represented by nitric oxide (NO) and adiponectin [82].

Multiple risk factors cumulate their effects. The presence of two risk factors increases the risk almost four times; if there are three risk factors, the rate of myocardial infarction increases seven times. Also, the level of exposure at risk factors determines considerable variations in the evolution of the atherosclerotic process and this is the reason why and early determination through different methods would be extremely useful in the evaluation of the cardiovascular risk [83]. Atherosclerosis and its consequences may develop in the absence of any risk factor, even in people who have a healthy life and without an apparent genetic predisposition [16].

In accordance with European Society of Cardiology Guidelines on Cardiovascular Disease Prevention (2007), the population should follow the next formula: 0 3 140 5 3 0, which suggest crucial measurements in keeping the cardiovascular health: without smoking (0), walking 3 km per day or 30 min of moderate activity (3), systolic pressure less than 140 mmHg (140), total cholesterol under 5 mmol/L (5), LDL-cholesterol under 3 mmol/L (3), eviction of obesity and diabetes (0) [84]. Actual guides recommend performing moderate physical activity minimum 30 min per day five times a week [85].

Epidemiologic data show that there are some hemostatic, thrombolytic and inflammation markers that are potential predictors of the risk for major atherosclerotic events, including myocardial infarction and stroke. These markers are related to fibrinolysis (e.g.: PAI 1—plasminogen activator inhibitor 1) or inflammation (CRP—C-reactive protein). PAI-1 plays an important role in cardiovascular diseases, mostly by inhibiting t-PAC (tissue plasminogen activator) [16, 86]. Inflammation biomarkers, especially CRP and lipoprotein-associated A2 phospholipase, are considered not only as potential risk predictors for stroke but also as prognostic factors [87]. CRP is considered to be a new proatherogenic inflammatory adipocytokine. CRP is an acute phase reactant, being synthesized mostly by the liver and regulated by circulating levels of IL6, IL1 and TNF-α. Recent studies demonstrated that high sensitive CRP is not only an atherosclerotic inflammatory marker but also a disease progression mediator, contributing to the formation and progression of the atheromatous plaque by promoting inflammation, thrombogenesis and modulatory endothelial function [88]. CRP induces the expression of adhesion molecule, selectins and MCP1 in endothelial cellular cultures, by increasing secretion of ET1 and IL6, and also stimulating angiotensin II action over receptors. By inhibiting NO endothelial secretions, CRP diminishes basal production and stimulated production of endothelial NO. CRP effect is potentiated by hyperglycemia and diminished by thiazolidinedione, an insulin sensitizer agent. CRP may also amplify proinflammatory activity of other adipokines, for example, PAI-1 intervention in the suppression of fibrinolysis and thrombogenesis by the inhibition of the activated plasminogen [89]. Increased plasmatic levels of PAI-1 are directly correlated with the cardiovascular risk and type 2 diabetes development. Even if platelets and endothelial cells represent a major source of PAI-1, in men, adipose tissue produces, also, PAI-1. Increased plasmatic levels of PAI-1 are found in obese patients and decrease with lowering weight [90].

Latest advances confirmed the role of Lp-PLA2 in advanced coronary disease evolution, being an important linking factor between lipid homeostasis and vascular inflammatory response. Selective inhibition of Lp-PLA2 reduces the development of the inner core atheroma and leads to plaque stabilization [91]. A lipoprotein is a lipid fraction that looks like an independent risk factor for atherosclerosis. It represents a modified LDL-cholesterol that has a characteristic protein fragment covalent linked to apo B and named apo(a), with an polymorphism and a structural analogy with the plasmatic plasminogen. Also, it has a complex prothrombotic action. Thus, Lp(a) seems to make the connection between atherosclerosis and thrombosis, the two processes being tightly related in atherosclerosis evolution [16, 92].

Serum amyloid A is an acute phase reactant, like CRP, that has been associated with systemic inflammation, related to the atherosclerosis process and used as a predictor for coronary disease and for cardiovascular prognosis. Levels of serum amyloid A are significantly correlated to insulin resistance and obesity in type 2 diabetes patients. Adipose tissue maintains amyloid at low levels in normal conditions, but an excess of it seems to stimulate this reactant. Serum amyloid A replaces apolipoprotein 1 from HDL-cholesterol, increasing the macrophage bond HDL and decreasing the cardioprotective HDL [81].

TNF-α is an inflammatory cytokine, which is released in high levels by obese patients and those with an increased insulin resistance, and contributes to the initiation and development of the atherosclerotic lesions. TNF-α activates the NF-κB nuclear factor transcription that accelerates the experimental atherosclerosis, partly by inducing the adhesion molecular expression, MCP-1 and E-selectin, in vascular smooth muscle cells and aortic endothelium. TNF-α reduces the bioavailability of nitric oxide in endothelial cells and modifies the endothelial-dependent vasodilatation, promoting its dysfunction; in addition of these effects, it might also induce apoptosis in endothelial cells [81].

Epidemiological research showed an obviously different frequency of atherosclerosis between geographic regions. The explanations are related to physicochemical properties of the drinking water and the meteorological factors. Oligoelements as calcium, magnesium, manganese, lithium, zinc, chrome and fluorine have proven antiatherogenic properties. It is known that the chronic absence of some oligoelements from the drinking water, with a consecutive decrease of its hardness is accompanied by an increase of the cardiovascular disease frequency. The opposite is the plumb excess and mostly the cadmium excess, which characterizes the soft water. Meteorological factors do not seem to be implied in the mechanism of the disease development. However, they represent important indicators of a major coronary accident occurrence, on an atherosclerotic fond [93].

Socioeconomical factors also increase the atherogen risk among the population: overstrain in the work place, physical and intellectual overexertion, sudden and frequent changes in the way of life and work, commuting, increased professional and familial responsibilities, conflictual states (familial, professional), social unintegration, irrational use of food, sedentary state, alcohol and excessive smoking. These situations are usually accompanied by an increased level of catecholamines, plasmatic lipids and blood pressure, which involves an intensified aggression over heart vessels [94].

An efficient therapeutic strategy presumes not only obtaining regression or retreat of existing atheroma but also modulating vascular impact in the beginning. It is important to mention the fact that atherosclerosis is one of the most frequent vascular disease in developed countries.

It is well known that the negative effect of high blood pressure over atherosclerosis needs a critical level of circulating lipoproteins [95]. However, antihypertensive treatment effects on atherosclerotic fond are not sufficiently known. Decoding the complex cellular and molecular mechanisms of atherogenesis process might certainly influence the therapeutic choice. Even if it has been tried on numerous ways to reduce LDL-cholesterol, there are a whole series of cardiovascular disease that cannot be efficiently treated. Starting from some medication that is centered over HDL, this promotes some certain antiatherogenic effects: antioxidative, anti-inflammatory, antithrombosis and endothelial stabilization [96].

Considering atherosclerosis as a disease with inflammatory substrate, in the acute phase HDL (that normally is anti-inflammatory) may become proinflammatory. Reactive species of oxygen generate an enzymatic system that can modify phospholipids and sterols by oxidation, reducing the HDL-cholesterol protection capacity against the unwanted oxidative changes at the molecular level [97].

Some experimental studies suggest that the use of mimetic peptides, such as apolipoprotein A-1, is capable of removing the oxidative products from lipoproteins and cellular membranes, giving back the normal structure and function of HDL-cholesterol [98]. In order to correct the HDL value, we currently use two classes of compounds: fibric acid derivatives and niacin derivatives. Dyslipidemia is considered as one of the main atherosclerotic risk factors and represents one of the atherogenic therapeutic targets [99].

Modern studies posit the therapy with cardiovascular cells (by exogenous ingestion or by an endogenous cellular mobilization) as effective in preventing and treating atherosclerotic lesions. Using bone marrow cells or autolog skeletal myoblasts in the beginning, it could be observed the fact that cardiac regeneration is produced through a variable repopulation accompanied by adjacent revascularization. Nowadays, the mesenchymal stem cells have large-scale utilization because of the immunosuppressant capacity and the ability to locate in the damaged tissue areas. The ability of stem cells to form myocardial cells has been studied both in vivo and in vitro research [100, 101]. Cardiomyoplasty is already used as a regeneration method of the damaged myocardium, using different cellular types [102]. This myocardial reconstructive technique, which is under a clinical evaluation and a rigorous immunological monitorization, could change the approach of cardiovascular disease therapy in the near future.

Author details

Elena Cojocaru[1], Alexandra Mastaleru[2*], Bogdan Tamba[3], Raluca Vasile[4], Razvan Cosmin Tudor[5], Carmen Valerica Ripa[6], Roxana Cobzaru[6] and Maria Magdalena Leon[2]

*Address all correspondence to: alexandra.mastaleru@gmail.com

1 "Gr.T.Popa" University of Medicine and Pharmacy, Discipline of Morphopathology, Iasi, Romania

2 "Gr.T.Popa" University of Medicine and Pharmacy, Discipline of Medical Semiology, Iasi, Romania

3 "Gr.T.Popa" University of Medicine and Pharmacy, Discipline of Pharmacology, Iasi, Romania

4 Psychiatrist in Sf. Nicolae Psychiatric Hospital, Roman, Romania

5 Orthopedic Surgeon in Regional Hospital of Vaslui, Romania

6 "Gr. T. Popa" University of Medicine and Pharmacy, Discipline of Parasitology, Iasi, Romania

References

[1] Poredos P, Jezovnik MK. Does the preventive effect of different drugs depend on location of the atherosclerotic process? International Angiology. 2008;**27**(4):274-280

[2] Fuster V. Chronic multivessel disease: Past, present and future. Rev Esp Cardiol. 2008;**61**(Suppl 2):2-9

[3] Rizzo M, Rizvi AA, Rini GB, Berneis K. The therapeutic modulation of atherogenic dyslipidemia and inflammatory markers in the metabolic syndrome: What is the clinical relevance? Acta Diabetologica. 2009;**46**(1):1-11. DOI: 10.1007/s00592-008-0057-4

[4] Segers D, Weinberg P, Krams R. Atherosclerosis: Cell biology and lipoproteins--shear stress and inflammation in plaque formation: New evidence. Current Opinion in Lipidology. 2008;**19**(6):627-628. DOI: 10.1097/MOL.0b013e328318db32

[5] Moreno PR, Sanz J, Fuster V. Promoting mechanisms of vascular health: Circulating progenitor cells, angiogenesis, and reverse cholesterol transport. Journal of the American College of Cardiology. 2009;**53**(25):2315-2323. DOI: 10.1016/j.jacc.2009.02.057

[6] Lamon BD, Hajjar DP. Inflammation at the molecular interface of atherogenesis: An anthropological journey. American Journal of Pathology. 2008;**173**(5):1253-1264. DOI: 10.2353/ajpath.2008.080442

[7] Rafieian-Kopaei M, Setorki M, Doudi M, Baradaran A, Nasri H. Atherosclerosis: Process, indicators, risk factors and new hopes. International Journal of Preventive Medicine. 2014;**5**(8):927-946

[8] ESHRE Capri Workshop Group. Hormones and cardiovascular health in women. Human Reproduction Update. 2006;**12**(5):483-497. DOI: 10.1093/humupd/dml028

[9] Butcovan D, Mocanu V, Baran D, Ciurescu D, Tinica G. Assessment of vulnerable and unstable carotid atherosclerotic plaques on endarterectomy specimens. Experimental and Therapeutic Medicine. 2016;**11**(5):2028-2032. DOI: 10.3892/etm.2016.3096

[10] Phillips LS, Langer RD. Postmenopausal hormone therapy: Critical reappraisal and a unified hypothesis. Fertility and Sterility. 2005;**83**(3):558-566. DOI: 10.1016/j.fertnstert.2004.11.012

[11] Marjoribanks J, Farquhar C, Roberts H, Lethaby A, Lee J. Long-term hormone therapy for perimenopausal and postmenopausal women. Cochrane Database of Systematic Reviews. 2017;**1**:CD004143. DOI: 10.1002/14651858.CD004143.pub5

[12] World Health Organization. Global Health Observatory (GHO) data [Internet]. Available from: http://www.who.int/gho/mortality_burden_disease/en/

[13] Sawabe M, Arai T, Kasahara I, Hamamatsu A, Esaki Y, Nakahara K et al. Sustained progression and loss of the gender-related difference in atherosclerosis in the very old: A pathological study of 1074 consecutive autopsy cases. Atherosclerosis. 2006;**186**(2):374-379. DOI: 10.1016/j.atherosclerosis.2005.07.023

[14] Chan MY, Woo KS, Wong HB, Chia BL, Sutandar A, Tan HC. Antecedent risk factors and their control in young patients with a first myocardial infarction. Singapore Medical Journal. 2006;**47**(1):27-30

[15] Anderson RE, Pfeffer MA, Thune JJ, McMurray JJ, Califf RM, Velazquez E et al. High-risk myocardial infarction in the young: The VALsartan In Acute myocardial iNfarcTion (VALIANT) trial. American Heart Journal. 2008;**155**(4):706-711. DOI: 10.1016/j.ahj.2007.11.016

[16] Kumar V, Abbas A, Aster J. Robbins & Cotran Pathologic Basis of Disease. 9th ed. Elsevier Philadelphia; 2015. 1408 p

[17] ESHRE Capri Workshop Group. Venous thromboembolism in women: A specific reproductive health risk. Human Reproduction Update. 2013;**19**(5):471-482. DOI: 10.1093/humupd/dmt028

[18] Liu S, Rouleau J, Joseph KS, Sauve R, Liston RM, Young D et al. Epidemiology of pregnancy-associated venous thromboembolism: A population-based study in Canada. Journal of Obstetrics and Gynaecology Canada. 2009;**31**(7):611-620

[19] Atsma F, Bartelink ML, Grobbee DE, van der Schouw YT. Postmenopausal status and early menopause as independent risk factors for cardiovascular disease: A meta-analysis. Menopause. 2006;**13**(2):265-279. DOI: 10.1097/01.gme.0000218683.97338.ea

[20] Archer DF. Premature menopause increases cardiovascular risk. Climacteric. 2009;**12** (Suppl 1):26-31

[21] Lobo RA. Menopause and stroke and the effects of hormonal therapy. Climacteric. 2007;**10**(Suppl 2):27-31. DOI: 10.1080/13697130701550903

[22] Shufelt CL, Bairey Merz CN. Contraceptive hormone use and cardiovascular disease. Journal of the American College of Cardiology. 2009;**53**(3):221-231. DOI: 10.1016/j.jacc.2008.09.042

[23] Grundy SM, Hansen B, Smith SC Jr, Cleeman JI, Kahn RA, American Heart Association, et al. Clinical management of metabolic syndrome: Report of the American Heart Association/National Heart, Lung, and Blood Institute/American Diabetes Association conference on scientific issues related to management. Arteriosclerosis, Thrombosis, and Vascular Biology. 2004;**24**(2):e19–e24. DOI: 10.1161/01.ATV.0000112379.88385.67

[24] Talayero BG, Sacks FM. The role of triglycerides in atherosclerosis. Current Cardiology Reports. 2011;**13**(6):544-552. DOI: 10.1007/s11886-011-0220-3

[25] Daniels TF, Killinger KM, Michal JJ, Wright RW Jr, Jiang Z. Lipoproteins, cholesterol homeostasis and cardiac health. International Journal of Biological Sciences. 2009;**5** (5):474-488

[26] Hausenloy DJ, Yellon DM. Targeting residual cardiovascular risk: Raising high-density lipoprotein cholesterol levels. Heart. 2008;**94**(6):706-714. DOI: 10.1136/hrt.2007.125401

[27] Cardenas GA, Lavie CJ, Cardenas V, Milani RV, McCullough PA. The importance of recognizing and treating low levels of high-density lipoprotein cholesterol: A new era in atherosclerosis management. Reviews in Cardiovascular Medicine. 2008;**9**(4):239-258

[28] Fernandez ML, Volek JS. Guinea pigs: A suitable animal model to study lipoprotein metabolism, atherosclerosis and inflammation. Nutrition & Metabolism (London). 2006;**27**(3):17. DOI: 10.1186/1743-7075-3-17

[29] Kapur NK, Musunuru K. Clinical efficacy and safety of statins in managing cardiovascular risk. Vascular Health and Risk Management. 2008;**4**(2):341-353

[30] Nesto RW. Beyond low-density lipoprotein: Addressing the atherogenic lipid triad in type 2 diabetes mellitus and the metabolic syndrome. American Journal of Cardiovascular Drugs. 2005;**5**(6):379-387

[31] Kim HS, Lee H, Park B, Park S, Kim H, Lee SH et al. Comparative analysis of the efficacy of low- and moderate-intensity statins in Korea. International Journal of Clinical Pharmacology & Therapeutics. 2016;**54**(11):864-871. DOI: 10.5414/CP202332

[32] Li Z, Tao Y, Huang J, Wang Q, Zhang DH, Wu XY. The characteristics of high density lipoprotein cholesterol and the relationship between high density lipoprotein cholesterol and the severity of coronary artery lesions in young men with acute myocardial infarction. Zhonghua Yi Xue Za Zhi. 2013;**93**(19):1458-1462

[33] Stone NJ, Robinson J, Lichtenstein AH, Merz CNB, Blum CB, Eckel RH et al. ACC/AHA guideline on the treatment of blood cholesterol to reduce atherosclerotic cardiovascular risk in adults. Circulation. 2013. DOI: 10.1161/01.cir.0000437738.63853.7a

[34] Velja-Asimi Z, Burekovic A, Dujic T, Dizdarevic-Bostandzic A, Semiz S. Incidence of prediabetes and risk of developing cardiovascular disease in women with polycystic ovary syndrome. Bosnian Journal of Basic Medical Sciences. 2016;**16**(4):298-306. DOI: 10.17305/bjbms.2016.1428

[35] Sim SY, Chin SL, Tan JL, Brown SJ, Cussons AJ, Stuckey BG. Polycystic ovary syndrome in type 2 diabetes: Does it predict a more severe phenotype? Fertility and Sterility. 2016;**106**(5):1258-1263. DOI: 10.1016/j.fertnstert.2016.06.040

[36] Apridonidze T, Essah PA, Iuorno MJ, Nestler JE. Prevalence and characteristics of the metabolic syndrome in women with polycystic ovary syndrome. Journal of Clinical Endocrinology and Metabolism. 2005;**90**(4):1929-1935. DOI: 10.1210/jc.2004-1045

[37] Dahlgren E, Johansson S, Lindstedt G, Knutsson F, Odén A, Janson PO et al. Women with polycystic ovary syndrome wedge resected in 1956 to 1965: A long-term follow-up focusing on natural history and circulating hormones. Fertility and Sterility. 1992;**57**(3):505-513

[38] Hudecova M, Jan H, Christian B, Poromaa Inger S. Long-term reproductive and metabolic consequences of PCOS. Current Diabetes Reviews. 2012;**8**(6):444-451

[39] Zhao L, Zhu Z, Lou H, Zhu G, Huang W, Zhang S et al. Polycystic ovary syndrome (PCOS) and the risk of coronary heart disease (CHD): A meta-analysis. Oncotarget. 2016;**7**(23):33715-33721. DOI: 10.18632/oncotarget.9553

[40] Pierpoint T, McKeigue PM, Isaacs AJ, Wild SH, Jacobs HS. Mortality of women with polycystic ovary syndrome at long-term follow-up. Journal of Clinical Epidemiology. 1998;**51**(7):581-586

[41] Wild S, Pierpoint T, McKeigue P, Jacobs H. Cardiovascular disease in women with polycystic ovary syndrome at long-term follow-up: A retrospective cohort study. Clinical Endocrinology. 2000;**52**(5):595-600

[42] Jordan WM, Anand JK. Pulmonary embolism. Lancet. 1961;**278**(7212):1146-1147. DOI: 10.1016/S0140-6736(61)91061-3

[43] Samson ME, Adams SA, Merchant AT, Maxwell WD, Zhang J, Bennett CL et al. Cardiovascular disease incidence among females in South Carolina by type of oral contraceptives, 2000-2013: A retrospective cohort study. Archives of Gynecology and Obstetrics. 2016;**294**(5):991-997. DOI: 10.1007/s00404-016-4143-5

[44] Catena C, Novello M, Lapenna R, Baroselli S, Colussi G, Nadalini E et al. New risk factors for atherosclerosis in hypertension: Focus on the prothrombotic state and lipoprotein (a). Journal of Hypertension. 2005;**23**(9):1617-1631

[45] Bönner G, Gysan DB, Sauer G. Prevention of arteriosclerosis. Importance of the treatment of arterial hypertension. Zeitschrift für Kardiologie. 2005;**94**(Suppl 3):56-65. DOI: 10.1007/s00392-005-1308-9

[46] Shklovskii BL, Prokhorchik AA, Koltunov AN, Lishchuk AN, Ryzhman NN, Ivanov AV et al. Myocardial infarction in young population. Voenno-Meditsinskiĭ Zhurnal. 2015;**336**(3):38-46

[47] Pérez de Isla L, Alonso R, Mata N, Saltijeral A, Muñiz O, Rubio-Marin P et al. Coronary heart disease, peripheral arterial disease, and stroke in familial hypercholesterolaemia: Insights from the SAFEHEART registry (Spanish Familial Hypercholesterolaemia Cohort Study). Arteriosclerosis, Thrombosis, and Vascular Biology. 2016;**36**(9):2004-2010. DOI: 10.1161/ATVBAHA.116.307514

[48] Davignon J. Apolipoprotein E and atherosclerosis. Beyond lipid effect. Arteriosclerosis, Thrombosis, and Vascular Biology. 2005;**25**(2):267-269. DOI: 10.1161/01.ATV.0000154570.50696.2c

[49] Bennet AM, Di Angelantonio E, Ye Z, Wensley F, Dahlin A, Ahlbom A et al. Association of apolipoprotein E genotypes with lipid levels and coronary risk. JAMA. 2007;**298**(11):1300-1311. DOI: 10.1001/jama.298.11.1300

[50] Heide S, Manfred K, Gläser C, Schulz S. Apolipoprotein E (apoE) polymorphism: A risk factor for fatal coronary sclerosis? Forensic Science International. 2009;**192**(1-3):62-66. DOI: 10.1016/j.forsciint.2009.07.020

[51] Nürnberger J, Kribben A, Philipp T, Erbel R. Arterial compliance (stiffness) as a marker of subclinical atherosclerosis. Herz. 2007;**32**(5):379-386. DOI: 10.1007/s00059-007-3030-z

[52] Lacolley P, Challande P, Osborne-Pellegrin M, Regnault V. Genetics and pathophysiology of arterial stiffness. Cardiovascular Research. 2009;**81**(4):637-648. DOI: 10.1093/cvr/cvn353

[53] Yasmin, O'Shaughnessy KM. Genetics of arterial structure and function: Towards new biomarkers for aortic stiffness? Clinical Science (London). 2008;**114**(11):661-677. DOI: 10.1042/CS20070369

[54] Kingwell B, Boutouyrie P. Genetic influences on the arterial wall. Clinical and Experimental Pharmacology & Physiology. 2007;**34**(7):652-657. DOI: 10.1111/j.1440-1681.2007.04655.x

[55] Trzos E, Uznańska B, Rechciński T, Krzemińska-Pakuła M, Bugała M, Kurpesa M. Myocardial infarction in young people. Cardiology Journal. 2009;**16**(4):307-311

[56] Teo KK, Ounpuu S, Hawken S, Pandey MR, Valentin V, Hunt D,. Tobacco use and risk of myocardial infarction in 52 countries in the INTERHEART study: A case-control study. Lancet. 2006;**368**(9536):647-658. DOI: 10.1016/S0140-6736(06)69249-0

[57] Makita S, Matsui H, Naganuma Y, Abiko A, Tamada M, Nakamura M. Diabetic state as a crucial factor for impaired arterial elastic properties in patients with peripheral arterial disease. Atherosclerosis. 2010;**208**(1):167-170. DOI: 10.1016/j.atherosclerosis.2009.06.033

[58] Wright RJ, Frier BM. Vascular disease and diabetes: Is hypoglycaemia an aggravating factor? Diabetes/Metabolism Research and Reviews. 2008;**24**(5):353-363. DOI: 10.1002/dmrr.865

[59] Jia G, DeMarco VG, Sowers JR. Insulin resistance and hyperinsulinaemia in diabetic cardiomyopathy. Nature Reviews Endrocrinology. 2016;**12**(3):144-153. DOI: 10.1038/nrendo.2015.216

[60] Pessina AC. Target organs of individuals with diabetes caught between arterial stiffness and damage to the microcirculation. Journal of Hypertension – Supplement. 2007;**25**(1):S13–S18. DOI: 10.1097/01.hjh.0000271504.62325.a4

[61] Safar ME, Rizzoni D, Blacher J, Muiesan ML, Agabiti-Rosei E. Macro and microvasculature in hypertension: Therapeutic aspects. Journal of Human Hypertension. 2008;**22**(9):590-595. DOI: 10.1038/jhh.2008.43

[62] Agabiti-Rosei E. From macro- to microcirculation: Benefits in hypertension and diabetes. Journal of Hypertension – Supplement. 2008;**26**(3):S15–S19

[63] van Guldener C, Stehouwer CD. Homocysteine and large arteries. Advances in Cardiology. 2007;**44**:278-301. DOI: 10.1159/000096748

[64] Fernández-Miranda C, Paz M, Aranda JL, Núñez V, Gómez P, Díaz-Rubio P et al. Homocysteine and progression of carotid atherosclerosis in patients with coronary disease. Medicina Clínica (Barcelona). 2003;**121**(15):561-564

[65] Page JH, Ma J, Chiuve SE, Stampfer MJ, Selhub J, Manson JE et al. Plasma total cysteine and total homocysteine and risk of myocardial infarction in women: A prospective study. American Heart Journal. 2010;**159**(4):599-604. DOI: 10.1016/j.ahj.2009.12.037

[66] Park CS, Ihm SH, Yoo KD, Kim DB, Lee JM, Kim HY et al. Relation between C-reactive protein, homocysteine levels, fibrinogen, and lipoprotein levels and leukocyte and platelet counts, and 10-year risk for cardiovascular disease among healthy adults in the USA. American Journal of Cardiology. 2010;**105**(9):1284-1288. DOI: 10.1016/j.amjcard.2009.12.045

[67] Handzha IM. Viral infection, atherosclerosis, and ischemic heart disease. Likars'ka Sprava. 2001;(1):65-67

[68] Vorob'ev AA, Abakumova IuV. Role of viral-herpetic infections in the etiology of atherosclerosis: Clinical, virological and immunological evidence. Vestnik Rossiĭskoĭ Akademii Meditsinskikh Nauk. 2003;(4):3-10

[69] Grundtman C, Kreutmayer SB, Almanzar G, Wick MC, Wick G. Heat shock protein 60 and immune inflammatory responses in atherosclerosis. Arteriosclerosis, Thrombosis, and Vascular Biology. 2011;**31**(5):960-968. DOI: 10.1161/ATVBAHA.110.217877

[70] Ayada K, Yokota K, Kobayashi K, Shoenfeld Y, Matsuura E, Oguma K. Chronic infections and atherosclerosis. Clinical Reviews in Allergy & Immunology. 2009;**37**(1):44-48. DOI: 10.1007/s12016-008-8097-7

[71] Lunardi C, Dolcino M, Peterlana D, Bason C, Navone R, Tamassia N et al. Endothelial cells' activation and apoptosis induced by a subset of antibodies against human cytomegalovirus: Relevance to the pathogenesis of atherosclerosis. PLoS One. 2007;**2**(5):e473. DOI: 10.1371/journal.pone.0000473

[72] Mehta JL. Inflammatory and Infectious Basis of Atherosclerosis. Basel, Boston, Berlin: Birkhauser; 2001. 267 p

[73] Pasqui AL, Bova G, Maffei S, Auteri A. Immune factors in atherosclerosis. Annali Italiani di Medicina Interna. 2005;**20**(2):81-89

[74] Wang YN, Che SM, Ma AQ. Clinical significance of serum cytokines IL-1beta, sIL-2R, IL-6, TNF-alpha, and IFN-v in acute coronary syndrome. Chinese Medical Sciences Journal. 2004;**19**(2):120-124

[75] Ozeren A, Aydin M, Tokac M, Demircan N, Unalacak M, Gurel A et al. Levels of serum IL-1beta, IL-2, IL-8 and tumor necrosis factor-alpha in patients with unstable angina pectoris. Mediators of Inflammation. 2003;**12**(6):361-365. DOI: 10.1080/09629350310001633360

[76] Nguyen JT, Myers N, Palaia J, Georgopoulos A, Rubins JB, Janoff EN. Humoral responses to oxidized low-density lipoprotein and related bacterial antigens after pneumococcal vaccine. Translational Research. 2007;**150**(3):172-179. DOI: 10.1016/j.trsl.2007.04.001

[77] Longo, Fauci, Kasper, Hauser, Jameson, Loscalzo. Harrison's Principles of Internal Medicine. 18th ed. The McGraw Hill Companies Inc. USA; 2012. 3611 p

[78] Ghandehari H, Le V, Kamal-Bahl S, Bassin SL, Wong ND. Abdominal obesity and the spectrum of global cardiometabolic risks in US adults. International Journal of Obesity. 2009;**33**(2):239-248. DOI: 10.1038/ijo.2008.252

[79] Wisse BE. The inflammatory syndrome: The role of adipose tissue cytokines in metabolic disorders linked to obesity. Journal of the American Society of Nephrology. 2004;**15**(11):2792-2800. DOI: 10.1097/01.ASN.0000141966.69934.21

[80] Berg AH, Scherer PE. Adipose tisue, inflammation, and cardiovascular disease. Circulation Research. 2005;**96**(9):939-949. DOI: 10.1161/01.RES.0000163635.62927.34

[81] Pischon T, Rimm EB. Adiponectine and risk of acute coronary syndrome: Defining the obesity phenotype. European Heart Journal. 2007;**28**(3):274-275. DOI: 10.1093/eurheartj/ehl454

[82] Cao H. Adipocytokines in obesity and metabolic disease. Journal of Endocrinology. 2014;**220**(2):T47–T59. DOI: 10.1530/JOE-13-0339

[83] Depairon M, Hayoz D, Darioli R. Early detection of atherosclerosis. Revue Médicale Suisse. 2006;**2**(51):330-332, 335-336

[84] Katić T, Sakić I, Bergovec M. Primary prevention of cardiovascular disease. Acta Medica Croatica. 2009;**63**(1):71-74

[85] Arias-Palencia NM, Solera-Martínez M, Gracia-Marco L, Silva P, Martínez-Vizcaíno V, Cañete-García-Prieto J et al. Levels and Patterns of Objectively Assessed Physical Activity and Compliance with Different Public Health Guidelines in University Students. PLoS One. 2015;**10**(11):e0141977. DOI: 10.1371/journal.pone.0141977

[86] Gils A. The pathophysiological relevance of PAI-1 in cardiovascular diseases and the development of monoclonal antibodies as PAI-1 inhibitors. Verhandelingen - Koninklijke Academie voor Geneeskunde van België. 2006;**68**(3):179-198

[87] Elkind MS. Inflammatory markers and stroke. Current Cardiology Reports. 2009;**11**(1):12-20

[88] Ridker PM, Silvertown JD. Inflammation, C-reactive protein, and atherothrombosis. Journal of Periodontology. 2008;**79**(8 Suppl):1544-1551. DOI: 10.1902/jop.2008.080249

[89] Khreiss T, József L, Potempa LA, Filep JG. Conformational rearrangement in C-reactive protein is required for proinflammatory actions on human endothelial cells. Circulation. 2004;**109**(16):2016-2022. DOI: 10.1161/01.CIR.0000125527.41598.68

[90] Martín-Timón I, Sevillano-Collantes C, Segura-Galindo A, Del Cañizo-Gómez FJ. Type 2 diabetes and cardiovascular disease: Have all risk factors the same strength? World Journal of Diabetes. 2014;**5**(4):444-470. DOI: 10.4239/wjd.v5.i4.444

[91] Wilensky RL, Macphee CH. Lipoprotein-associated phospholipase A2 and atherosclerosis. Current Opinion in Lipidology. 2009;**20**(5):415-420. DOI: 10.1097/MOL.0b013e3283307c16

[92] Gudnason V. Lipoprotein (a): A causal independent risk factor for coronary heart disease? Current Opinion in Cardiology. 2009;**24**(5):490-495. DOI: 10.1097/HCO.0b013e32832f0a5b

[93] Ong CN, World Health Organization. Water Sanitation Health [Internet]. Available from: http://www.who.int/water_sanitation_health/dwq/nutrientschap5.pdf

[94] Duvigneaud N, Wijndaele K, Matton L, Deriemaeker P, Philippaerts R, Lefevre J et al. Socio-economic and lifestyle factors associated with overweight in Flemish adult men and women. BMC Public Health. 2007;**7**:23. DOI: 10.1186/1471-2458-7-23

[95] Remaley AT, Amar M, Sviridov D. HDL-replacement therapy: Mechanism of action, types of agents and potential clinical indications. Expert Review of Cardiovascular Therapy. 2008;**6**(9):1203-1215. DOI: 10.1586/14779072.6.9.1203

[96] Meyers CD, Kashyap ML. Pharmacologic elevation of high-density lipoproteins: Recent insights on mechanism of action and atherosclerosis protection. Current Opinion in Cardiology. 2004;**19**(4):366-373

[97] Shah PK. Focus on HDL: A new treatment paradigm for athero-thrombotic vascular disease. Expert Opinion on Investigational Drugs. 2000;**9**(9):2139-2146. DOI: 10.1517/13543784.9.9.2139

[98] Van Lenten BJ, Navab M, Anantharamaiah GM, Buga GM, Reddy ST, Fogelman AM. Multiple indications for anti-inflammatory apolipoprotein mimetic peptides. Current Opinion in Investigational Drugs. 2008;**9**(11):1157-1162

[99] Navab M, Reddy ST, Van Lenten BJ, Anantharamaiah GM, Fogelman AM. The role of dysfunctional HDL in atherosclerosis. Journal of Lipid Research. 2009;**50**(Suppl):S145–S149. DOI: 10.1194/jlr.R800036-JLR200

[100] Christoforou N, Gearhart JD. Stem cells and their potential in cell-based cardiac therapies. Progress in Cardiovascular Diseases. 2007;**49**(6):396-413. DOI: 10.1016/j.pcad.2007.02.006

[101] Grosser N, Schröder H. Therapy with NO donors-antiatherogenic and antioxidant actions. Herz. 2004;**29**(1):116-122. DOI: 10.1007/s00059-004-2530-3

[102] Lamb EK, Kao GW, Kao RL. Cellular cardiomyoplasty: Its past, present, and future. Methods in Molecular Biology. 2013;**1036**:1-17. DOI: 10.1007/978-1-62703-511-8_1

Chapter 4

Cardiovascular Risk Assessment in Developing World

Parinya Chamnan and Wichai Aekplakorn

Additional information is available at the end of the chapter

http://dx.doi.org/10.5772/intechopen.69041

Abstract

Many international and national authorities recommend that cardiovascular risk assessment using multivariate risk scores be used to identify individuals at high risk of cardiovascular disease (CVD). This approach is likely to assure that resources in developing countries are allocated to those who need it most. However, not many developing countries have implemented this approach and different countries have varying progresses in adopting the concept. While many developing countries solely described estimated cardiovascular risk by applying existing CVD risk scores to their population's cross-sectional data, a number of countries have validated and recalibrated existing risk scores and only a few have developed new risk scores specific to their populations. To enhance the adoption of such a policy in developing countries, new CVD risk prediction charts for low- and medium-resource settings were developed and endorsed by the WHO and International Society of Hypertension. However, a number of issues need to be addressed, including development of population-specific risk scores, recalibration of available risk scores and uncertainty over cost-effectiveness of CVD risk assessment in developing countries. Although this high risk approach might represent an effective and practical strategy for developing countries, a complementary population-based approach is also needed to maximize benefits for CVD prevention.

Keywords: cardiovascular disease, risk assessment, prediction, primary prevention, developing countries

1. Introduction

Quantitative assessment of cardiovascular risk has become part of strategies for prevention of cardiovascular disease (CVD) in many countries [1, 2]. Many international and national authorities have recommended that cardiovascular risk assessment using multivariate risk scores be used to identify individuals at high risk of cardiovascular disease, to whom preventive interventions can be targeted [3–6]. This high-risk approach has been advocated and routinely used in many developed countries [7, 8]. However, it has not been frequently used in developing countries. This chapter summarizes evidence on cardiovascular risk assessment in developing countries by (i) describing the overall rationale for using cardiovascular risk scores; (ii) systematically reviewing the literature on cardiovascular risk scores that have been developed, validated and/or practically used in developing countries; (iii) exploring issues surrounding the utility of the cardiovascular risk scores in these countries; and (iv) limitations and implications for alternative approaches.

2. Concept and rationale for cardiovascular risk assessment

Observational studies have shown a positive continuous association between traditional cardiovascular risk factors and CVD risk [9–11]. For example, results from the Prospective Studies Collaboration, a meta-analysis of almost 900,000 healthy men and women in 61 prospective observational studies, show a linear, continuous relationship between serum total cholesterol and the risk of death from ischemic heart disease. Similar associations were also held true for each of other traditional risk factors such as blood sugar [10] and blood pressure [11]. This underlines the importance of efforts to address each individual risk factor for prevention of cardiovascular disease.

However, there is evidence that clustering of risk factors confers higher levels of CVD risk than each individual risk factor. Evidence from observational prospective studies suggests that a small effect of an individual risk factor on CVD risk could be magnified in the presence of other risk factors [10, 12, 13]. In other words, an individual with mildly abnormal levels of several risk factors often has a greater absolute CVD risk than someone with a raised level of one risk factor. For example, data from the EPIC-Norfolk cohort revealed that CVD risk could vary up to 30-fold in people with the same levels of traditional CVD risk factors, such as cholesterol and blood pressure, but different abnormalities in other risk factors [10] (**Figure 1**).

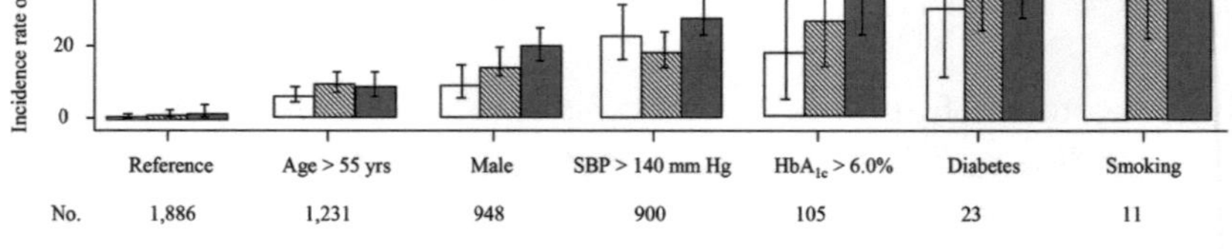

Figure 1. Absolute rates of cardiovascular events over 10 years in individuals with different levels of CVD risk factors in EPIC-Norfolk [10] (n = 10,144), Reference group: non-smoking women aged ≤ 55 years with a SBP of ≤ 140 mm Hg and an HbA_{1c} ≤ 6.0%, *$p < 0.001$, Reproduced with approval from Diabetologia.

The combined effect of risk factors on absolute risk of CVD underlines the importance of using multivariate risk prediction tools.

Randomized controlled trials have confirmed that treatment with lipid-lowering medication reduces the risk of ischemic heart disease and stroke, regardless of pre-treatment blood cholesterol levels or other characteristics of the study participants. Overall, there was a 19% reduction in coronary mortality for each 1 mmol/L reduction of low density lipoprotein (LDL) cholesterol [14]. Similarly, trial evidence suggests that blood pressure-lowering drugs reduce the risk of developing CVD events with comparable relative risk reductions at different pre-treatment levels of blood pressure [15]. This suggests that substantial benefits could be achieved from modifying these risk factors at any starting level in individuals whose absolute CVD risk is high for whatever aetiological reason. The concept of treating individuals with a disease diagnosed by a threshold of one single risk factor, e.g. diabetes, hypertension or hypercholesterolemia, has thus been challenged [12, 16].

Key question is how we can identify those at high CVD risk, which preventive interventions could be targeted. Compelling evidence points out that absolute risk assessment, based on the combined effect of multiple risk factors, is likely to be an approach of choice. Compared with multifactorial CVD risk assessment, major CVD risk factors such as blood pressure or blood lipid levels are, individually, poorer predictors of future CVD risk and of the benefits of treatment in individuals with and without existing CVD [1, 10, 16]. In addition, primary prevention informed by multifactorial CVD risk assessment is likely to prevent a similar number of cardiovascular events at a possibly lower cost than a single-factor approach [17].

There are a number of reasons why it may be important to quantify the risk of developing cardiovascular disease (**Table 1**). The clear rationale for the development of a risk score is critical to how its validity is assessed and how it is used.

First, risk scores may be used to rank individuals and groups according to their absolute cardiovascular risk so that preventive interventions for those at greatest risk could be targeted [1, 7]. Concerning this purpose, it is the ranking that is important and not necessarily the absolute risk estimates. The ranking of absolute CVD risk is clearly essential for making collective decisions about treatment and preventive interventions in the population. This is rather important for the government/public health professionals, whose decision-making will be done based on such information alongside careful consideration on costs incurred and possible harms from screening and subsequent preventive interventions.

Additionally, risk assessment is also used as a tool to provide prognostic information or estimation of the possible absolute benefits from therapeutic/preventive interventions. In this case, accurate estimation of the absolute risk is crucial. An estimate of absolute CVD risk can inform the potential for absolute risk reduction, which provides patients with an idea of expected benefit from a therapy or intervention. This is more relevant to individual, rather than collective, decision-making. However, further research is needed to understand the process by which the clinician and patient interact once cardiovascular risk has been assessed. Providing CVD risk estimates to doctors and patients may improve perceived CVD risk and

Rationale	Examples of utility of cardiovascular risk assessment in practice
Risk stratification	To rank individuals according to CVD risk and identify those at high risk for preventive interventions
	The Government makes decision if providing preventive intervention to a certain proportion of the population is affordable and acceptable.
Prognostication	To provide prognostic information to an individual, e.g. an individual is informed about how likely he/she will develop cardiovascular disease in the next 10 years
	To provide possible absolute benefits from therapeutic/preventive interventions, e.g. a doctor can discuss with his/her patients about to what extent that their CVD risk will reduce if they adhere to treatment and achieve certain therapeutic goals
Primary prevention	To motivate an individual to modify health behaviours or adhere to treatment, i.e. when a patient know smoking and high cholesterol contributes much to increased CVD risk, he/she may be more encouraged to stop smoking, adopt healthy diet or regularly take statins
	Monitoring CVD risk over time, e.g. information on favourable changes in absolute CVD risk after an individual has adopted a healthy lifestyle will help enhance adherence to such a lifestyle.

Table 1. Overall rationale for cardiovascular risk assessment.

medical prescribing particularly in high-risk groups [18]; however, there is no strong evidence that a CVD risk assessment performed by a clinician helps to improve CVD-related health outcomes [8].

Finally, the principle justification for calculating cardiovascular risk as part of a preventive strategy is to motivate individuals to adhere to favourable behaviour modification and medical treatments. Apparently, two unchangeable risk factors, age and sex, contribute most to the predictive value of a CVD risk score. However, it may be difficult to persuade patients to change their behaviour using CVD risk scores that are mostly driven by risk factors that they cannot change. Risk scores which incorporate modifiable risk factors may be more useful for preventive strategies. That is, it may be important to use risk scores comprised of modifiable risk factors rather than using a score dominated by fixed parameters [7]. This approach is of particular interest as lifestyle risk factors, such as inadequate physical activity, poor dietary habits and adiposity, have been reported to deteriorate blood pressure, serum cholesterol and glucose-insulin homeostasis and also associated with novel cardiovascular risk factors such as endothelial function and inflammatory markers[19].

3. Development and utility of CVD risk scores in developing countries

Although cardiovascular risk assessment is recommended by many authorities, it has not been widely and routinely implemented in developing countries. This may be explained by a number of reasons. First, a small number of existing risk scores were originally developed in developing countries. Most CVD risk scores were derived from European descent populations in developed countries, whose background CVD risk may be significantly different from that in developing countries. For example, CVD risk scores developed in a relatively high-risk population, such as Framingham risk equations, will overestimate the absolute risk when applied to a novel population with a lower background CVD risk [20]. This phenomenon emphasizes that recalibration should be done before using such a risk score in a new population. However, a few developing countries have carried out recalibration of available risk scores partly because a small number of prospective cohorts are available in these countries and populations. Further, there is still debate over the cost-effectiveness of implementation of such an approach in developing countries. This may have affected policy decision concerning cardiovascular risk assessment in these resource-constrained countries.

A different approach was taken to overcome problems regarding the validity of using available risk scores in a novel population in developing countries. Using epidemiologic survey data from the Comparative Risk Assessment Project and the Asia Pacific Cohort Studies Collaboration, the WHO and International Society of Hypertension (ISH) developed CVD risk prediction charts specific to low- and medium-resource countries in 14 different WHO sub-regions, based on age, sex, systolic blood pressure, presence of type 2 diabetes mellitus, smoking status and total serum cholesterol levels (**Figure 2**) [21, 22]. They also developed a non-laboratory-based version of the risk prediction charts, which can be used in settings where measurement of blood cholesterol is not feasible.

Developing countries have different progresses in adopting the concept of cardiovascular risk assessment (**Table 2**). Some developing countries have only applied existing risk scores, namely Framingham risk equations, SCORE and WHO/ISH CVD risk prediction charts,

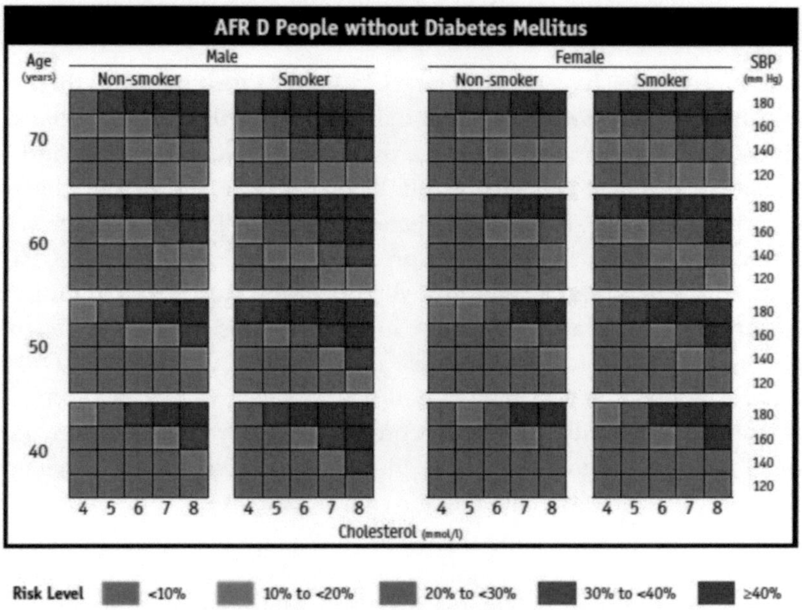

Figure 2. WHO/ISH risk prediction chart for Africa Sub-region D, 10-year risk of a fatal or non-fatal cardiovascular event by gender, age, systolic blood pressure, total blood cholesterol and smoking status in people without diabetes, Reproduced with approval from the WHO [22].

Describing estimated CVD risk and the burden of high CVD risk in its population	Validation and recalibration of existing risk scores in its population	Developing a new CVD risk score specific to its population
Saudi Arabia, Mozambique, Jamaica, Pakistan, Sri Lanka Nepal, Mongolia, Cambodia	Greece, Iran, Czech Republic, Poland, Lithuania, Russia	China, Thailand, Malaysia

Table 2. Examples of developing countries that have adopted concept of cardiovascular risk assessment.

to cross-sectional risk factor data to obtain estimated CVD risk and describe the burden of high absolute CVD risk in the population. For example, low prevalences of high CVD risk according to the WHO/ISH CVD risk prediction charts were observed in many developing countries such as Saudi Arabia, Nigeria, Iran, Pakistan, Nepal, Sri Lanka and Cambodia, with lower than 10% of the populations being considered high CVD risk [21, 23].

Other countries carried out a validation study to see if the existing risk scores performed well in predicting cardiovascular events in its population and further recalibrated the risk scores [24–26]. For example, the office-based Framingham risk equations were recalibrated in 46,674 participants in the Golestan Cohort in North-East of Iran and the authors found that the risk score performed reasonably well in predicting CVD mortality (aROC of 0.76–0.79) and overestimated CVD risk in men [25]. The SCORE was validated against CVD mortality in Central and Eastern Europe and former Soviet Union countries, using prospective data from the WHO MONICA project and HAPIEE study. In the MONICA cohort, the SCORE showed only moderate discriminatory ability (aROC of 0.54–0.69) and good calibration in Czech Republic, Poland and Lithuania, but overestimation of fatal CVD in Russia [26].

A few developing countries have derived new CVD risk scores specific to their populations; these include China, Thailand and Malaysia. Using data on 9903 men and women participating in the USA-PRC Collaborative Study of Cardiovascular Epidemiology Cohort, a new CVD risk score was developed based on age, systolic blood pressure, serum total cholesterol, body mass index, current smoking status and diabetes mellitus [27]. The risk score was validated in another large Chinese cohort with good predictive ability. In Thailand, CHD risk score was developed using data from a cohort of workers of the Electric Generating Authority of Thailand, [28] and this multivariate risk score has been endorsed to use in patients with and without diabetes, and a simpler approach using presence or absence of CVD risk factors is recommended for population screening. Based on cost-effectiveness evidence, cardiovascular risk assessment using multivariate risk scores has recently been endorsed as part of the Universal Health Coverage Benefit Package [29]. However, there is no clear evidence about to what extent this approach has been adopted in clinical practice.

4. Issues surrounding the utility of CVD risk scores

Cardiovascular risk scores have been widely used in Western countries for almost 20 years and were introduced at a time when the cost of cholesterol-lowering drugs was an important political issue. International and national recommendations have specified cardiovascular risk thresholds that are considered justification for prescribing therapy. As these figures were based largely on the proportion of the population requiring treatment and the total cost of treatment, it is therefore uncertain if all health systems, particularly in developing countries, can afford such a policy.

4.1. Laboratory- versus non-laboratory-based CVD risk assessment

While most CVD risk assessment tools were based on a set of cardiovascular risk factors including laboratory factors such as cholesterol, a number of risk scores including simple or routinely available risk factors may be more relevant and applicable to developing countries, where laboratory testing is unavailable. Of note, it has been demonstrated in many studies that laboratory- and non-laboratory-based CVD risk assessments are similarly effective at predicting future cardiovascular disease [30–32]. A modelling study based on data from the EPIC-Norfolk cohort and published evidence on effectiveness of key preventive interventions clearly suggests that inviting individuals at high risk identified using routine data for a vascular risk assessment could prevent a similar number of new cardiovascular events with potential cost-saving, compared to inviting all individuals for laboratory-based CVD risk assessment [33]. Cost-effectiveness analyses confirm that single-stage or multi-stage non-laboratory-based CVD risk assessment had a more attractive cost-effectiveness ratio or ICER than a laboratory-based Framingham risk-based approach, as reflected by lower estimated costs and higher QALYs [34].

4.2. Are population-specific risk scores needed?

The most commonly used cardiovascular risk score was originally developed in 5,573 men and women participating in the Framingham study in the early 1970s, which generally performs well in North America, but have reportedly performed less well in other populations. An alternative to attempting to find a universal risk score that will work in all populations may be to develop or recalibrate population-specific risk assessment tools.

Is it worth developing a new risk score which best suits with a new population or trying to improve the ability of the existing risk score to predict future disease events by including novel risk factors? The answer is likely to be 'No' for developing countries. Developing a new CVD risk score for developing countries or recalibrating existing risk scores in these countries may not be practical as it requires a prospective cohort to develop and validate the risk equations. A lack of prospective cohorts in developing countries will also limit the opportunities to recalibrate the existing risk scores in these countries/populations. Furthermore, including novel risk factors, such as biomarkers or genetic information, to a risk score with traditional CVD risk factors adds little to the predictive ability at disproportionately considerable costs [35, 36]. This may be too expensive for clinical practice in both developed and developing countries. Furthermore, there is rarely evidence that reductions in any of these novel markers will lower cardiovascular risk [37]. Therefore, rather than attempting to develop a new risk assessment tool, it may be more beneficial to make sure that existing risk assessment tools are used more broadly and routinely throughout clinical practice.

However, there remains a paradox of practice concerning CVD risk assessment in developing countries. While a population specific CVD risk score may be needed, a lack of prospective cohorts in developing countries prevent them from recalibrating available risk scores or developing a new one. While emphasis should be put on using existing risk scores more broadly and routinely, these risk scores seem to perform poorly in the developing countries and may lead to misclassification of individuals who do and do not require treatments.

4.3. Is universal CVD risk assessment in developing countries cost-effective?

As screening for high-risk individuals using CVD risk scores always comes with costs related to screening itself and subsequent preventive interventions, whether it is cost-effective in settings of resource-scarce countries is an important concern. With limited resources, it might be sensible to focus preventive efforts on those who will benefit most. Furthermore, the ratio of costs to benefits will be more favourable in individuals where the benefits are larger and this approach usually leads to manageable numbers of individuals.

CVD risk stratification will enable the government to use resources in a highly efficient way. Different thresholds for starting intensive preventive interventions may be applied to countries with different resources. For example, the WHO recommends that a 10-year CVD risk threshold of 30–40% may be used in medium- and low-resource countries [38]. When applying a WHO-ISH CVD risk prediction charts to randomly selected individuals from a number of developing countries such as Nigeria, Iran, China, Pakistan, Georgia, Nepal, Cuba and Sri Lanka, adopting WHO recommended 30% CVD risk threshold would help reduce healthcare expenditure by avoiding unnecessary drug treatment and thus reducing drug costs [21]. As equipment and facilities for CVD risk screening in developing countries may be limited, the WHO and International Society of Hypertension in 2002 proposed a simple approach to cardiovascular risk stratification based on history, blood pressure measurement and selective urine analysis for those with systolic/diastolic blood pressure of ≥140/90 mmHg [39]. Also, the WHO proposed different scenarios of CVD risk management which may be suitable to set with different diagnostic and therapeutic facilities and resources (**Table 3**).

However, it remains uncertain if universal CVD risk screening is cost-effective for resource-constrained settings in developing countries. In Thailand, cardiovascular risk assessment using a population-specific risk score is recommended for men and women aged 35 years and above at five-year intervals. The corresponding budget impact analysis shows that such an approach was financially feasible for the Thai setting, with the incremental cost-effectiveness ratio below the country's ceiling threshold of USD 4530/QALY [29]. In the contrary, a modelling study in Malaysian population suggests that universal screening would result in screening an additional 7169 individuals, with an incremental cost of USD 115,033 for detection of one additional high-risk individual in comparison to targeted screening of those aged 35 years and above [40]. Further, incremental cost and impact of detection of high-risk individuals would be higher for women than men for both universal screening and screening specific age groups. The authors suggested that targeted gender- and age-specific screening strategies would ensure more optimal use of limited resources compared to the country's policy recommendations of universal screening [40].

Resource availability	Scenario 1	Scenario 2	Scenario 3
Human resource	Non-physician health workers	Medical doctor or specially trained nurse	Medical doctor with access to full specialist care
Equipment	Stethoscope, blood pressure measurement device, measuring tape or weighing scale Optional: test tubes, holder, burner, solution or test strips for checking urine glucose	Stethoscope, blood pressure measurement device, tape and weighing scale, test tubes, holder, burner, solution or test strips for checking urine glucose and albumin	Stethoscope, blood pressure measurement device, tape and weighing scale, electrocardiograph, ophthalmoscope, urine analysis, blood analysis: fasting blood sugar, electrolytes, creatinine, cholesterol and lipoproteins
Generic drugs	Essential: thiazide diuretics Optional: metformin (for refill)	Thiazide diuretics, Beta blockers, Angiotensin converting enzyme inhibitors, calcium channel blockers (sustained release formulations) (Reserpine and methyldopa if the above anti-hypertensives are unavailable), Aspirin, Metformin (for refill)	Thiazide diuretics, Beta blockers, Angiotensin converting enzyme inhibitors, calcium channel blockers (sustained release formulations) (Reserpine and methyldopa if the above anti-hypertensives are unavailable), Aspirin, Insulin, Metformin, Glibenclamide, Statins (if affordable) Angiotensin receptor blocker (if affordable)

Table 3. Three scenarios for CVD risk assessment for setting with different resource availability, adapted from WHO CVD risk management package for low and medium resource settings [38].

4.4. Preventive interventions following CVD risk assessment

There are challenges concerning preventive interventions following CVD risk assessment. Different preventive interventions, ranging from lifestyle modification to medication, are recommended for individuals or groups with different levels of absolute CVD risk. For example, healthy diet, adequate physical activity and weight control should be encouraged in all individuals, and monitoring of CVD risk profiles every 3-6 months, nicotine replacement therapy, giving statins in those with an absolute 10-year risk of ≥20%, and prescribing antiplatelet drugs in those with a 10-year risk of ≥30% [41]. However, there remains unclear whether such differential interventions can be implemented in developing countries, where basic infrastructure and resources for preventive interventions in primary care may be lacking.

5. Limitations and implications for alternative approaches

Although identifying individuals or groups at high risk using multivariate CVD risk scores is beneficial, the 'population-based' strategy, which aims at reducing risk in the entire population, regardless of each individual's level of risk and potential benefits, may also be needed. Ability of CVD risk scores to identify individuals at high risk is a key to effective high-risk strategies. It may be more effective to concentrate our efforts and resources where the need, and therefore the benefit, is likely to be greatest. Interventions are also matched well with the needs of individuals, probably resulting in better motivation and compliance to medications or behaviour change [42]. However, the benefits of the high-risk approach are limited to a minority of the population. Further, a high-risk strategy demands that individuals change eating, smoking and physical activity habits that may be largely shaped and constrained by social norms (e.g. to eat differently from family and friends), and may thus be seen as 'behaviourally inappropriate'. As this approach does not seek to address the underlying causes of health problems in the population, it is only palliative and temporary [43]. The high-risk approach was described by Geoffrey Rose as 'no more than an expensive rescue operation, offering disappointingly little towards solving the overall problem', so it cannot be the sole means for prevention of cardiovascular disease [42].

Given compelling evidence that more cases of cardiovascular disease arise from a larger number of people at low risk than the smaller number of people at high risk, it might be more beneficial to shift the whole distribution of risk factors, such as body mass index, cholesterol or blood glucose, in the population in a favourable direction (population-based strategy). This phenomenon is commonly observed for diseases where the association of the disease with risk factors is linear or curvilinear, while the population distribution of these risk factors is approximately normal. For example, Emberson et al. demonstrated that small reductions in the population distribution of cardiovascular risk factors (total cholesterol and systolic blood pressure) might prevent similar or more CVD events than a strategy focusing preventive efforts on those at highest risk [44]. Therefore, in addition to a high-risk approach, there may be an important role for a 'population-based approach' to shift the population distribution of CVD risk factors.

In practice, balanced implementation of the high-risk and population-based approaches for CVD prevention is likely to be necessary [2]. Within resource-constrained health service systems in developing countries, the high-risk preventive strategies, which focus efforts on those at highest risk, may be seen as a feasible and cost-effective means of prevention. However, complementary population-based preventive strategies are also needed to address the cause of the disease incidence in the population.

In conclusion, CVD risk stratification in developing countries will assure that limited resource be allocated to individuals or groups who need it most. In developing countries, the clear rationale for cardiovascular risk assessment is crucial. The main rationale for cardiovascular risk assessment includes ranking individuals according to absolute cardiovascular risk for the purpose of targeting therapy to those at greatest risk, providing prognostic information or accurate estimation of the likely benefits from preventive/therapeutic interventions, and motivating individuals to change their behaviours and adhere to treatments. As not many developing countries have adopted this approach, a number of issues need to be addressed, including development of population-specific risk scores, recalibration of available risk scores and uncertainty over cost-effectiveness of CVD risk assessment in developing countries. Although this high-risk approach appears to be effective and practical for developing countries, a complementary population-based approach is needed to maximize benefits for CVD prevention.

http://dx.doi.org/10.5772/intechopen.69041

Author details

Parinya Chamnan[1]* and Wichai Aekplakorn[2]

*Address all correspondence to: parinya.chamnan@cardiomet-res.org

1 Cardiometabolic Research Group, Department of Social Medicine, Sanpasitthiprasong Hospital,Ubon Ratchathani, Thailand

2 Department of Community Medicine, Faculty of Medicine, Ramathibodi Hospital, Mahidol University, Bangkok, Thailand

References

[1] Lloyd-Jones DM. Cardiovascular risk prediction: Basic concepts, current status, and future directions. Circulation. 2010;**121**(15):1768-1777

[2] Hingorani AD, Psaty BM. Primary prevention of cardiovascular disease: Time to get more or less personal? Journal of the American Medical Association. 2009;**302**(19):2144-2145

[3] Piepoli MF, Hoes AW, Agewall S, Albus C, Brotons C, Catapano AL, et al. 2016 European Guidelines on cardiovascular disease prevention in clinical practice: The sixth joint task force of the european society of cardiology and other societies on cardiovascular disease prevention in clinical practice (constituted by representatives of 10 societies and by invited experts) developed with the special contribution of the european association for cardiovascular prevention & rehabilitation (EACPR). European Heart Journal. 2016;**37**(29):2315-2381

[4] Prepared by JBS 2. Joint British Societies' guidelines on prevention of cardiovascular disease in clinical practice. Heart. 2005;**91**(Suppl 5):v1-v52

[5] Prepared by Third report of the national cholesterol education program (NCEP). Expert panel on detection, evaluation, and treatment of high blood cholesterol in adults (Adult Treatment Panel III) final report. Circulation. 2002;**106**(25):3143-3421

[6] Goff Jr, DC, Lloyd-Jones DM, Bennett G, Coady S, D'Agostino RB, Gibbons R, et al. 2013 ACC/AHA guideline on the assessment of cardiovascular risk: A report of the American College of Cardiology/American Heart Association Task Force on practice guidelines. Circulation. 2014;**129**(25 Suppl 2):S49-S73

[7] Chamnan P, Simmons RK, Sharp SJ, Griffin SJ, Wareham NJ. Cardiovascular risk assessment scores for people with diabetes: A systematic review. Diabetologia. 2009;**52**(10):2001-2014

[8] Brindle P, Beswick A, Fahey T, Ebrahim S. Accuracy and impact of risk assessment in the primary prevention of cardiovascular disease: A systematic review. Heart. 2006;**92**(12):1752-1759

[9] Prospective Studies Collaboration, Lewington S, Whitlock G, Clarke R, Sherliker P, Emberson J. et al. Blood cholesterol and vascular mortality by age, sex, and blood pressure: A meta-analysis of individual data from 61 prospective studies with 55,000 vascular deaths. Lancet. 2007;**370**(9602):1829-1839

[10] Chamnan P, Simmons RK, Jackson R, Khaw KT, Wareham NJ, Griffin SJ. Non-diabetic hyperglycaemia and cardiovascular risk: Moving beyond categorisation to individual interpretation of absolute risk. Diabetologia. 2011;**54**(2):291-299

[11] Lewington S, Clarke R, Qizilbash N, Peto R, Collins R, Prospective Studies C. Age-specific relevance of usual blood pressure to vascular mortality: A meta-analysis of individual data for one million adults in 61 prospective studies. Lancet. 2002;**360**(9349):1903-1913

[12] Jackson R, Lawes CM, Bennett DA, Milne RJ, Rodgers A. Treatment with drugs to lower blood pressure and blood cholesterol based on an individual's absolute cardiovascular risk. Lancet. 2005;**365**(9457):434-441

[13] Neaton JD, Wentworth D. Serum cholesterol, blood pressure, cigarette smoking, and death from coronary heart disease. Overall findings and differences by age for 316,099 white men. Multiple risk factor intervention trial research group. Archives of Internal Medicine. 1992;**152**(1):56-64

[14] Baigent C, Keech A, Kearney PM, Blackwell L, Buck G, Pollicino C, et al. Efficacy and safety of cholesterol-lowering treatment: Prospective meta-analysis of data from 90,056 participants in 14 randomised trials of statins. Lancet. 2005;**366**(9493):1267-1278

[15] Yusuf S, Sleight P, Pogue J, Bosch J, Davies R, Dagenais G. Effects of an angiotensin-converting-enzyme inhibitor, ramipril, on cardiovascular events in high-risk patients. The heart outcomes prevention evaluation study investigators. The New England Journal of Medicine. 2000;**342**(3):145-153

[16] Jackson R. Cardiovascular risk prediction: are we there yet? Heart. 2008;**94**(1):1-3

[17] Ndindjock R, Gedeon J, Mendis S, Paccaud F, Bovet P. Potential impact of single-risk-factor versus total risk management for the prevention of cardiovascular events in Seychelles. Bulletin of the World Health Organization. 2011;**89**(4):286-295

[18] Usher-Smith JA, Silarova B, Schuit E, Moons KG, Griffin SJ. Impact of provision of cardiovascular disease risk estimates to healthcare professionals and patients: A systematic review. British Medical Journal Open. 2015;**5**(10):e008717

[19] Mozaffarian D, Wilson PW, Kannel WB. Beyond established and novel risk factors: lifestyle risk factors for cardiovascular disease. Circulation. 2008;**117**(23):3031-3038

[20] Liu J, Hong Y, D'Agostino RB, Sr, Wu Z, Wang W, Sun J, et al. Predictive value for the Chinese population of the Framingham CHD risk assessment tool compared with the Chinese multi-provincial cohort study. Journal of the American Medical Association. 2004;**291**(21):2591-2599

[21] Mendis S, Lindholm LH, Anderson SG, Alwan A, Koju R, Onwubere BJ, et al. Total cardiovascular risk approach to improve efficiency of cardiovascular prevention in resource constrain settings. Journal of Clinical Epidemiology. 2011;**64**(12):1451-1462

[22] Mendis S, Lindholm LH, Mancia G, Whitworth J, Alderman M, Lim S, et al. World Health Organization (WHO) and International Society of Hypertension (ISH) risk prediction charts: Assessment of cardiovascular risk for prevention and control of cardiovascular disease in low and middle-income countries. Journal of Hypertension. 2007;**25**(8):1578-1582

[23] Otgontuya D, Oum S, Buckley BS, Bonita R. Assessment of total cardiovascular risk using WHO/ISH risk prediction charts in three low and middle income countries in Asia. BMC Public Health. 2013;**13**:539

[24] Panagiotakos DB, Georgousopoulou EN, Fitzgerald AP, Pitsavos C, Stefanadis C. Validation of the HellenicSCORE (a Calibration of the ESC SCORE Project) regarding 10-Year risk of fatal cardiovascular disease in Greece. Hellenic Journal of Cardiology. 2015;**56**(4):302-308

[25] Sepanlou SG, Malekzadeh R, Poustchi H, Sharafkhah M, Ghodsi S, Malekzadeh F, et al. The clinical performance of an office-based risk scoring system for fatal cardiovascular diseases in North-East of Iran. PLoS One. 2015;**10**(5):e0126779

[26] Vikhireva O, Pajak A, Broda G, Malyutina S, Tamosiunas A, Kubinova R, et al. SCORE performance in Central and Eastern Europe and former Soviet Union: MONICA and HAPIEE results. European Heart Journal. 2014;**35**(9):571-577

[27] Wu Y, Liu X, Li X, Li Y, Zhao L, Chen Z, et al. Estimation of 10-year risk of fatal and nonfatal ischemic cardiovascular diseases in Chinese adults. Circulation. 2006;**114**(21):2217-2225

[28] Yamwong S. Development of Thai CVD risk score. Public Health Foundation and Thailand Research Funds, Bangkok. 2005

[29] Teerawattananon Y, Kingkaew P, Koopitakkajorn T, Youngkong S, Tritasavit N, Srisuwan P, et al. Development of a health screening package under the universal health coverage: The role of health technology assessment. Health Economics. 2016;**25**(Suppl 1):162-178

[30] Gaziano TA, Young CR, Fitzmaurice G, Atwood S, Gaziano JM. Laboratory-based versus non-laboratory-based method for assessment of cardiovascular disease risk: The NHANES I follow-up study cohort. Lancet. 2008;**371**(9616):923-931

[31] D'Agostino RB, Sr., Vasan RS, Pencina MJ, Wolf PA, Cobain M, Massaro JM, et al. General cardiovascular risk profile for use in primary care: The Framingham heart study. Circulation. 2008;**117**(6):743-753

[32] Chamnan P, Simmons RK, Hori H, Sharp S, Khaw KT, Wareham NJ, et al. A simple risk score using routine data for predicting cardiovascular disease in primary care. British Journal of General Practice. 2010;**60**(577):e327-e334

[33] Chamnan P, Simmons RK, Khaw KT, Wareham NJ, Griffin SJ. Estimating the population impact of screening strategies for identifying and treating people at high risk of cardiovascular disease: Modelling study. British Medical Journal. 2010;**340**:c1693

[34] Pandya A, Weinstein MC, Salomon JA, Cutler D, Gaziano TA. Who needs laboratories and who needs statins?: Comparative and cost-effectiveness analyses of non-laboratory-based, laboratory-based, and staged primary cardiovascular disease screening guidelines. Circulation: Cardiovascular Quality and Outcomes. 2014;**7**(1):25-32

[35] Lippi G, Salvagno GL, Targher G, Guidi GC. Multiple biomarkers for the prediction of first major cardiovascular events and death: Considerable costs and limited benefits. Medscape General Medicine. 2007;**9**(1):34

[36] Wang TJ, Gona P, Larson MG, Tofler GH, Levy D, Newton-Cheh C, et al. Multiple biomarkers for the prediction of first major cardiovascular events and death. The New England Journal of Medicine. 2006;**355**(25):2631-2639

[37] Ridker PM, Brown NJ, Vaughan DE, Harrison DG, Mehta JL. Established and emerging plasma biomarkers in the prediction of first atherothrombotic events. Circulation. 2004;**109**(25 Suppl 1):IV6-IV19

[38] Wolrd Health Organization. WHO CVD-risk management package for low- and medium resource settings. Switzerland: Wolrd Health Organization; 2002

[39] Chalmers J, World Health Organization International - Society of H. Enhancing risk stratification in hypertensive subjects: How far should we go in routine screening for target organ damage? Journal of Hypertension. 2002;**20**(7):1255-1257

[40] Selvarajah S, Haniff J, Kaur G, Guat Hiong T, Bujang A, Chee Cheong K, et al. Identification of effective screening strategies for cardiovascular disease prevention in a developing country: Using cardiovascular risk-estimation and risk-reduction tools for policy recommendations. BMC Cardiovascular Disorders. 2013;**13**:10

[41] World Health Organization. Prevention of cardiovascular disease: Guidelines for assessment and managemnet of cardiovascular risk. Geneva: World Health Organization; 2007

[42] Rose G. Rose's strategy of preventive medicine. New York: Oxford University Press; 2008

[43] Rose G. Sick individuals and sick populations. International Journal of Epidemiology. 2001;**30**(3):427-432; discussion 33-34

[44] Emberson J, Whincup P, Morris R, Walker M, Ebrahim S. Evaluating the impact of population and high-risk strategies for the primary prevention of cardiovascular disease. European Heart Journal. 2004;**25**(6):484-491

Chapter 5

Cardiovascular Disease and Diabetes: Two Sides of the Same Coin!

Sayeeda Rahman, Md. Anwarul Azim Majumder,
Russell Kabir, Mainul Haque, Subir Gupta,
Sana Mohammad Yasir Arafat, Nkemcho Ojeh and
Prasad Dalvi

Additional information is available at the end of the chapter

http://dx.doi.org/10.5772/intechopen.69038

Abstract

Cardiovascular disease (CVD) and type 2 diabetes (T2DM) are rapidly rising around the globe. Empirical researches demonstrated rapid increase in mortality and morbidity related to CVD and T2DM. Much of the diabetes-associated morbidity and mortality predominantly reflects its deleterious effect on macrovascular and microvascular diseases. The microvascular complications of T2DM include retinopathy, neuropathy and nephropathy and the macrovascular complications include ischemic heart disease, cerebrovascular disease and peripheral vascular diseases. Research indicates that coronary heart disease (CHD) is the major cause of mortality in people with T2DM. Herein, this chapter reviews relationship between CVD and T2DM, associated complications and effectiveness of relevant treatment modalities to treat/prevent diabetic macrovasculopthy. Macrovascular disease occur due to underlying obstructive atherosclerotic changes of major arteries which cause functional and structural abnormalities of blood vessels. The long-term complications can be controlled and prevented by controlling glycemia, maintaining normal lipid profiles, adopting a healthy lifestyle and using pharmacological interventions. Clinical trials have shown that lifestyle interventions help in prevention and reduction of CVD risk, but evidence for long-term CVD outcomes is lacking. A multidisciplinary approach involving patients, health professionals and researchers and governments should be undertaken to reduce the incidence and prevalence of diabetes-related cardiovascular complications.

Keywords: cardiovascular diseases, type 2 diabetes, vasculopathy, macrovascular diseases, atherosclerosis, pathophysiology, pathogenesis

1. Introduction

Cardiovascular disease (CVD) is the major cause of morbidity and mortality in people with type 2 diabetes (T2DM) [1, 2], and coronary heart disease (CHD) is the most common cause of death among people with T2DM. It is estimated that up to 80% of the 200 million people suffering with T2DM globally die of CVD every year [3, 4]. In recent years, the pandemic of T2DM has emerged as a major and growing health problem. The cardiovascular (CV) complications associated with T2DM cause a considerable amount of disability, premature mortality, loss of productivity and tremendously increase burden on health care systems and economies worldwide [5–7]. Among the major complications, the development of CVD is two to four times higher in people with T2DM as compared with people without the condition [8, 9]. Thus, CVD and T2DM have become inseparable which need to be addressed by the global health initiatives.

T2DM acts as an independent risk factor for several forms of CVD (micro- and macrovascular diseases), and people with T2DM are more likely to develop CVD due to a variety of risk factors [10]. Preclinical manifestations of macrovascular diseases are developed much earlier in newly diagnosed, never-treated T2DM patients [11], and such macrovascular changes are also observed even in normoglycemic and normotensive offspring of parents with T2DM [12, 13]. Furthermore, early manifestations of preclinical vasculopathy and development of macrovascular disease were potentially found to be at increased risk with impaired glucose tolerance (IGT) [13]. The CV complications of T2DM have a significant impact on individuals, families, health systems, and economic development worldwide [14]. According to the International Federation of Diabetes, $673 billion was spent on diabetes in 2015 which is 12% of global health expenditure [15]. It is imperative to control the initiators of vasculopathy that ultimately develop into long-term CV complications by adopting a healthy lifestyle and using pharmacological interventions. This chapter reviews relationship between CVD and T2DM, associated complications and relevant treatment modalities to treat/prevent diabetic macrovasculopthy.

2. Cardiovascular disease risk in diabetes

CVD are the number one cause of death globally – more people die annually from CVD than from any other cause. Individuals at risk of CVD may demonstrate hypertension, hyperglycemia, and hyperlipidemia as well as overweight and obesity. According to World Health Organization [16]:

- Approximately 17.5 million people died worldwide from CVDs in 2012, representing 31% of all deaths.
- Of all CVD deaths, an estimated 7.4 million were due to CHD and 6.7 million were due to stroke.
- An estimated 75% of CVD deaths take place in low- and middle-income countries.
- Of the 16 million deaths (≤70 years of age) as a result of non-communicable diseases 37% are caused by CVDs.

The main contributing factor in the increasing prevalence of CVD deaths is the increase in the cases of diabetes at very alarming rate, in particular, due to increasing prevalence of obesity, lifestyle choices, urbanization, aging, and genetic factors [17]. According to the International Diabetic Federation [15]:

- In 2015, 415 million people had diabetes, and in 2040, 642 million people will develop diabetes worldwide.
- At present, 3/4 of people with diabetes live in low and middle income countries.
- In 2015, 1 in 11 adults had diabetes, and in 2040, 1 in 10 adults will have diabetes.
- One in two adults with diabetes remains undiagnosed.
- Every 6 s 1 person dies from diabetes.
- Five million deaths occurred in 2015 as a result of diabetes.

3. Diabetes and macrovasculopthy: double trouble!

The alterations in vascular homeostasis that include anatomic, structural, and functional changes in blood vessels lead to multi-organ dysfunction and increase CV risk burden [18]. Diabetic microvascular and macrovascular complications have similar pathogenetic mechanisms and characteristics. The microvascular complications include retinopathy, neuropathy and nephropathy and the macrovascular complications include ischemic heart disease, cerebrovascular disease and peripheral vascular diseases [19–21].

The relationship between diabetes and CVD is complex and multifactorial [22]. Studies demonstrated the following macrovascular complications in T2DM patients:

- In diabetic men, CV mortality increased three-fold [23, 24] and in diabetic women, two to fivefold [25, 26].
- Patients with diabetes who develop clinical CVD have higher mortality than those CVD patients with no diabetes [26, 27].
- T2DM is considered to be one of the six major controllable risk factors for CVD [28].
- T2DM and IGT are related to increased risk of CV problems [28].
- People with T2DM also have high rates of hypertension, lipid abnormality, and obesity, which contribute to their high rates of CVD [28].
- T2DM is associated with increased risks of stroke, myocardial infarction, hypertension and intermittent claudication [29–31].
- Approximately 7% of people with T2DM have had a stroke at time of diagnosis and, indeed, stroke is the second major cause of death in T2DM [31].
- Risk of fatal stroke is increased 2–3-fold compared with non-diabetics [29], accounting for 15% of all deaths in T2DM [32].

- It was also demonstrated that 18% of diabetic patients have evidence of coronary heart disease at diagnosis, and the risk of a fatal myocardial infarction is increased 2–4 times in people with T2DM [29].
- Fatal cardiovascular events were 70 times more common than deaths from microvascular complications [33].
- Peripheral vascular disease (PVD) is estimated to be the most costly complication of diabetes in relation to inpatient care.
- PVD greatly increases the risk of intermittent claudication, foot ulcers, gangrene, infection and amputation [32].
- Lower extremity amputations are at least 10 times more common in people with diabetes than in non-diabetic individuals in developed countries and more than half of all non-traumatic lower limb amputations are due to T2DM [34].

4. Pathophysiology of diabetic macrovasculopathy

Atherosclerotic vascular disease mainly occurs due to endothelial dysfunction [35, 36], which is the failure of the vascular endothelium to subserve its normal role in vasodilatation and/or vascular homeostasis. The physiological impairment that causes diabetic vasculopathy includes endothelial dysfunction, platelet hyper-reactivity, smooth muscle cell (SMC) dysfunction, impaired fibrinolysis coupled with a tendency for thrombosis and coagulation, and increased inflammation [37, 38]. Endothelial dysfunction links each of these pathological manifestations to develop macrovasculopathy [39]. The main regulatory function of endothelium stimulation includes vasodilatation; other mechanisms include vasoconstriction, and antiplatelet and anticoagulant effects [40]. Endothelial dysfunction lead to morphologic and structural vascular changes [41]. Capillary endothelium rapidly disappears [42], intercellular junctions weaken causing increased vascular permeability [43], protein synthesis is dysregulated and expression of adhesion glycoproteins on endothelial cells is altered [42–45], thereby triggering adherence of monocytes and leucocytes and their increased transendothelial migration [43].

The characteristic feature of diabetic complications includes the progression of atherosclerotic lesion or alteration of vasculature, which is a major cause of CVD development [46]. It was shown that diabetes accelerates these processes by stimulating the atherogenic activity of vascular SMC and these considered as the integral part in the development of atherosclerosis [35]. The process begins as a response to chronic minimal injury to the endothelium leading to it being dysfunctional. Fewer vascular SMCs are also found in patients with diabetes with advanced atherosclerotic lesions [47]. Diabetes alters vascular smooth muscle function in ways that promote atherosclerotic lesion formation, plaque instability and clinical events. Platelet aggregation and adhesion are seen in diabetic patients [48–51]. The process involves an increase in intrinsic platelet activation and decrease endogenous inhibitors of platelet activity [35]. Platelets exhibit enhanced platelet aggregation activity in the early disease state that may precede the development of CVD [48–54]. T2DM also brings about some changes in coagulation of blood. A procoagulant state has been shown in people having diabetes [55–57]. It was demonstrated that there is an increase in plasminogen activator inhibitor-1 (PAI-1), von Willebrand factor (vWF), fibrinogen, factor VII and thrombin–antithrombin complexes in macrovascular diseases and poor glycemic control [55–61].

5. Pathogenesis of vasculopathy

It is now well-established that metabolic, humoral and hemodynamic factors contribute to the characteristic dysfunction in diabetic vasculopathy. Prolonged hyperglycemia is considered as a major factor in the pathogenesis of diabetic vasculopathy [62–64]. Hyperglycemia together with several other factors accelerates the progression of atherosclerosis. In particular, hypoglycemia increases oxidative stress [65]; enhances leucocyte–endothelial interaction [66], and glycation of protein, lipoproteins, apolipoproteins and clotting factors, which cumulatively enhance vasomotor tone, vascular permeability, growth and remodeling [42–45]. Moreover, hyperglycemia delays endothelial cell replication, increases cell death [42, 45, 67–70] and potentially accelerates the atherosclerotic process. Glucose-induced damage occurs through advanced glycation, activation of protein kinase C (PKC), and sorbitol accumulation [71, 72]. Early glycated products on collagen, intestinal tissues and blood vessels undergo a series of chemical rearrangement to form irreversible AGE. AGE product promotes atherosclerotic effect by receptor-mediated biological activities e.g. monocyte emigration, release of cytokines and growth factors from macrophages and increase in endothelial permeability and procoagulant activity [73].

Dysregulation of Lipid metabolism underlies pathogenesis of macrovascular diseases of diabetes origin [74]. Diabetic dyslipidemia causes increase in total cholesterol and low-density lipoprotein (LDL) and -decrease in high-density lipoprotein (HDL) and high triglyceride levels [74, 75]. LDL and other lipoproteins enter the endothelial cells by vascular transport and may get modified by oxidation, glycation, aggregation, association with proteoglycans or incorporation to immune-complexes [76–78].

Insulin resistance is a common feature associated with T2DM and development of CVDs. Insulin resistance precedes the development of overt T2DM and leads to endothelial dysfunction and increases blood plasma levels of endothelin and vWF [79]. Furthermore, insulin resistance may cause increase in arterial blood pressure by triggering several mechanisms, such as, activation of sympathetic nervous system, increase in renal sodium retention, alteration in transmembrane cation transport, augmentation of growth-promoting actions of SMCs and vascular hyperactivity [80–82].

Increased expression and action of various cytokines and growth factors in T2DM may induce macrovascular injury via activation of proliferative cytokines epidermal growth factor [83] and platelet-derived growth factor (PDGF) [84]. Metabolic and hemodynamic factors interact to stimulate the expression of cytokines and growth factors in the various vascular trees, which contribute to the characteristic dysfunction observed in diabetic vasculopathy [20].

Intracellular hyperglycemia has been implicated in the pathogenesis of diabetic complications through the activation of PKC, an intracellular second messenger system [85, 86]. PKC appears to be activated in a range of diabetic tissues including heart and aorta [20]. The beta isoform of PKC is involved in abnormalities of endothelial-dependent vasodilatation in diabetes by promoting superoxide ions (O_2^-) to react with nitric oxide to produce peroxynitrate ($ONOO^-$), which damages tissues and activates monocyte macrophages [87]. Diabetic vasculopathy is characterized by early migration of monocytes into the arterial wall [88]. Monocytes differentiate into macrophages to form foam cells which secrete growth factors and metalloproteinases. The growth factors stimulate cell proliferation and matrix production, and the metalloproteinases cause matrix degeneration [78].

Another major factor involved in the pathogenesis of vasculopathy is oxidative stress [89–91]. Increased oxidative stress in T2DM induces generation of free radicals that cause vascular tissue damage. In the pathogenesis of diabetic vasculopathy, white blood cells (WBCs) play a potential role. High WBC count predicts a decrease in insulin action and development of T2DM [92]. Inflammation is a primary risk factor for CVD [93], and proinflammatory cytokines and C-reactive protein are found to be linked to the development of diabetes. Increased WBC count, in particular, increase in activated neutrophils is a major contributing factor in development of CVD [94]. Activation of neutrophils leads to altered rheological properties of blood, increases blood corpuscular adhesion, and damages endothelium with cytotoxic reactive oxygen species and proteolytic enzymes [95]. These changes trigger activity of granulocytes and monocytes in endothelial injury site and result in atherogenesis. Besides, leucocyte adhesiveness/aggregation is found to be slightly increased in those who have had concomitant diabetes [96].

6. Diagnosis of vasculopathy

Increased arterial stiffness is a dysfunctional property of the arterial circulation that leads to CVD. The stiffening of aorta and other central arteries is a potential risk factor for increased CV morbidity and mortality [97]. Arterial stiffness can be measured by a number of methods. Some of these are more widely used in the clinical settings as these are simple, accurate and, reproducible and thus can easily be applied for the evaluation of CV risk. [98]. Most of them are complex or need sophisticated technical equipment, which limits their application in clinical practice. Among the non-invasive and simple methods of evaluating arteries, pulse wave velocity (PWV) [99] and augmentation index (AI) [100–103] measurement are widely used as indexes of large artery elasticity and stiffness.

Pulse wave velocity (PWV) is the oldest and probably the best clinical measure of stiffness over an arterial segment [104]. The technique of PWV is valid and reproducible, and has been widely applied in clinical and research setting [105]. PWV is determined by measurement of the time taken for the pulse wave to traverse the distance between two fixed measuring points [99]. PWV may be measured in various segments of the arterial circulation [106] and is therefore derived as (distance [m]/time [s]), in m/s, ranging from 5–20 m/s [104]. It is assessed either between carotid and femoral arteries (aortic PWV) or carotid and radial arteries known as brachial PWV [99].

http://dx.doi.org/10.5772/intechopen.69038

The pulse wave analysis (PWA) is the generation of ascending aortic pressure wave [107]. The system is used to assess central aortic pressure which depends on accurate recording of the radial pulse wave [108, 109]. The radial pressure pulse contains all the basic information from which the ascending aortic pulse is generated [107]. It is calibrated against the brachial pressure, then generation of ascending aortic pressure waveform through the use of generalized transfer function in a computerized process [107]. It gives information to ventricular/vascular interaction from both pressure and time values, as calculated from the synthesized aortic waveform. Therefore, PWA used for deriving central arterial pressure waveforms, from which *augmentation index* (AI) and the timing of the reflected pressure wave can be determined as indices of arterial stiffness. Aortic AI is defined as the increment in pressure after the first systolic shoulder to the peak of the aortic pressure expressed as a percentage of aortic pulse pressure [110]. It is a surrogate measure of systemic arterial stiffness [111–113] which is calculated from the derived aortic waveforms using PWA and expressed as a percentage (%).

Pulse pressure is one of the simplest measures of arterial stiffness, varies with the rigidity of the arterial wall and easily practicable in the clinical setting. Pulse pressure is the difference between systolic and diastolic BP, depends on cardiac output, large artery stiffness and wave reflection. It can be easily measured by sphygmomanometer. However, pulse pressure alone is inadequate to assess arterial stiffness accurately. Brachial pulse pressure may not change despite increasing arterial stiffness when induced by circulating angiotensin II [114].

Pulse contour analysis estimates arterial stiffness non-invasively and measures both capacitive (storage) and cushioning (oscillatory) arterial functions. In this technique arterial pulse contour is used to assess large artery capacitance and the capacitance of smaller arteries that are the primary source of reflected waves or oscillations in the arterial system. This technique involves tonometry at the radial artery, but the compliance is derived differently, using a model of the circulation and an assessment of diastolic pressure decay. Pressure pulse contour analysis requires estimation of cardiac output from an algorithm.

Photoplethysmography records the digital volume pulse [115]. This technique records the transmission of infrared light passing through the finger to measure the alteration in flow and produces a volume waveform. A stiffness index and a reflexion index that reflect systemic arterial stiffness are developed using this technique. The technique is relatively simple and easily portable [105]. However, problems include the damping of peripheral pulse, and temperature-dependant changes in the peripheral circulation.

Ultrasound and Doppler techniques are used to visualize wall thickness and vascular diameter on a monitor screen. Using an ultrasound transducer to perpendicularly project ultrasound beams to the artery, the optimal sound reflections from the wall are obtained and the reflected echoes from the wall and lumen are monitored. Simultaneously, blood pressure is also measured to adjust the change in arterial diameter to estimate arterial stiffness.

Magnetic resonance imaging (MRI) technique is used to measure vascular compliance and distensibility. The technique demonstrates the inverse relationship between aortic distensibility and age, i.e. aortic distensibility is reduced in hypertensive patients [116], and that arterial compliance is reduced in patients with CAD but increased in athletes [117].

Oscillometric BP measurement can be used to estimate the arterial stiffness. The pattern of oscillations depends on arterial stiffness. As the cuff is deflated, oscillations are increased, reaching a peak at mean arterial pressure. By coupling this to a computer algorithm, an index of arterial stiffness can be calculated.

7. Treatment modalities of diabetic vasculopathy

CVD is a major complication and the leading cause of early death among people with T2DM [118]. Much of the diabetes-associated morbidity and mortality predominantly reflects its deleterious effect on macrovascular and microvascular diseases [119, 120]. As T2DM is a complex metabolic disorder characterized by hyperglycemia, hypertension, hypercoagulability, and dyslipidemia, the diabetic patients with CVD require therapy for each of these metabolic abnormalities to reduce atherogenesis and prevent CV complications [121]. The main strategies for an effective therapy are to reverse insulin resistance, restore beta cell function, and control hepatic glucose output. The key treatment modalities include lifestyle modification and pharmacological interventions.

7.1. Lifestyle management

Lifestyle management is an essential part of management of T2DM and CVD in diabetic patients. Dietary restriction is recommended to achieve weight loss and reduce the risk factors for CVD in T2DM. Calorie restriction and weight loss bring down the blood pressure to normal limits and improves blood lipid profile, especially triglycerides and very low-density lipoprotein cholesterol. Exercise improves glycemic control, reduces certain CV risk factors, and increases psychological wellbeing [122]. In addition, physical training has been shown to reverse insulin resistance by increasing the number of skeletal muscle glucose transporters, which may reduce the need for hypoglycemic agents [123].

7.2. Pharmacotherapy

Patients with T2DM who do not show improvements in blood glucose levels with diet therapy are generally prescribed *oral hypoglycemic drugs*. These drugs control hyperglycemia by either increasing the release of insulin from the pancreatic beta cells or increasing the sensitivity of peripheral tissues to insulin [124–126]. The efficacy of these drugs depends on the endogenous capacity of insulin production in the T2DM patients. Among the main oral hypoglycemic drugs are biguanides and sulfonylureas. Other prominent groups include α-glucosidase inhibitors, meglitinides, thiazolidinediones, incretin mimetics, and dipeptidyl peptidase-4 (DPP-4) inhibitors.

Sulfonylureas act by promoting insulin secretion from the pancreatic islet beta cells and may improve insulin resistance in muscle and liver by improving insulin sensitivity in these target tissues. Metformin is the most commonly used biguanide and is suggested as the first-line drug of choice. It reduces hepatic glucose output, primarily by decreasing gluconeogenesis, and to a lesser extent, by enhancing insulin sensitivity in hepatic and peripheral tissues. Alpha-glucosidase inhibitors such as acarbose, miglitol, and voglibose inhibit the α-glucosidase enzyme which is essential for the release of glucose from more complex carbohydrates and is found in the brush border of enterocytes of small intestine. Thus, α-glucosidase inhibit the absorbance of carbohydrates in the gut and help in prevention of hyperglycemia [127]. Rosiglitazone and pioglitazone belong to the group of thiazolidinediones. The thiazolidinediones enhance insulin sensitivity in the peripheral target tissues such as muscle and adipose tissue, and inhibit hepatic glucose production to some extent, but have no effect on insulin secretion. When used in combination with other antidiabetic drugs, the thiazolidinediones achieve significant improvement in insulin resistance. Importantly, the thiazolidinediones have also been shown to improve the dyslipidemia in patients with T2DM.

A recent advance in the management of T2DM has been the development and clinical use of incretin-based therapies, i.e., glucagon-like peptide-1 (GLP-1) receptor analogs (e.g., exenatide) and DPP-4 inhibitors (e.g., sitagliptin, vildagliptin, saxagliptin) [128–131]. GLP-1 receptor agonists mimic the action of GLP-1 and increase the incretin effect in patients with T2DM, stimulating the release of insulin. DPP-4 inhibitors prevent degradation of endogenous GLP-1 and glucose-dependent insulinotropic polypeptide, thereby helping in glycemic control [129].

Anti-hypertensive drugs i.e. diuretics, angiotensin-converting enzyme (ACE) inhibitors, beta-blockers, angiotensin II receptor blockers, and calcium antagonists have been effectively used in the treatment of high blood pressure control. For the prevention of cardiovascular complications and treatment of hypertension these drugs have shown beneficial effects in T2DM patients. In such patients, thiazide diuretics have been found to be very effective either alone or in combination with other anti-hypertensive therapy [132]. ACE inhibitors have beneficial effects in reducing macrovascular complications, improving insulin sensitivity and glucose metabolism in T2DM patients [18, 133]. ACE inhibitors can be used alone, however, their effectiveness significantly increases when combined with a thiazide diuretic or other antihypertensive therapeutic drugs [132]. Calcium antagonists have been found to be beneficial in controlling hypertension when used as part of a combined regimen [132]. Anti-hypertensive therapy using a calcium channel blocker lowers the risks of developing complications associated with beta-blocker usage [134].

Lipid-lowering agents reduce the risk of major macrovascular events in patients with T2DM [135, 136]. Statins (HMG-CoA reductase inhibitors) are considered to be first-line therapy for the majority of T2DM patients [137] and has demonstrated benefit in both the primary and secondary prevention of CVD [135, 138, 139]. Several clinical studies have found beneficial effects associated with fibrate therapy [140–142]. Statins are effective in lowering plasma LDL-C, apolipoprotein B, and total cholesterol to HDL-C ratio, whereas fibrates are found to be beneficial in lowering triglycerides, shifting LDL particle size from smaller to larger, and raising HDL-C that results in lowering the total cholesterol to HDL-C ratio [18].

Anti-platelet drugs i.e. aspirin, clopidogrel, dipyridamole, and the glycoprotein IIb/IIIa receptor antagonists reduce CV risk in patients with T2DM [137] due to their antiplatelet effects. Aspirin irreversibly inhibits prostaglandin H synthase (cyclo-oxygenase-1) in platelets and megakaryocytes that prevents synthesis of thromboxane A2, which is a potent vasoconstrictor and platelet aggregant [143]. The thienopyridine derivatives, such as clopidogrel, ticlopidine, are converted to active metabolites in the liver which significantly decrease blood platelet activation via their action on the adenosine phosphate receptors on platelets. Dipyridamole increases cAMP concentration in platelets by inhibiting phosphodiesterase enzyme, and the increased cAMP levels inhibit activation of cytoplasmic second messengers. Dipyridamole also promotes prostacyclin release and inhibits thromboxane A2 synthesis. Glycoprotein IIb/IIIa receptor antagonists inhibit the final common pathway for platelet aggregation.

8. Clinical trials on prevention strategies and therapeutic approaches for diabetic vasculopathy

Growth of overweight and obese population due to diet and life-style changes worldwide correlates with the global T2DM epidemic [144]. However, majority of the studies focusing on diabetes prevention were not designed to assess CV outcomes [145]. There is a need for studies to explore the effect of exercise and diet on quality of life, morbidity, and mortality, with a special focus on CV outcomes.

Clinical trials examining the effect of *intensive glucose control* on CVD did not report consistency in beneficial effects of intensive glycemic control on CV events [146–149]. Although the risk of microvascular complications was reduced with strict glucose control in T2DM patients, its beneficial effects on CVD prevention or reduction remain ambiguous [150–152]. Data from UKPDS 34 (the United Kingdom Prospective Diabetes Study) suggested a protective effect of improved glucose control on CVD, CV mortality, and all-cause mortality [146]. However, a number of large randomized, controlled trials have reported conflicting results. ADVANCE (Action in Diabetes and Vascular Disease: Preterax and Diamicron Modified Release Controlled Evaluation) [147], VADT (Veterans Affairs Diabetes Trial) [153], and NAVIGATOR (Nateglinide and Valsartan in Impaired Glucose Tolerance Outcomes Research) [154] showed no effect of intensive glucose control on major CV events. However, ACCORD (Action to Control Cardiovascular Disease in Diabetes) [149] demonstrated an increased risk of death from CV causes and total mortality associated with intensive glucose control. In the PROactive (Prospective Pioglitazone Clinical Trial in Macrovascular Events) study [155], patients treated with pioglitazone had a significant 16% reduction in mortality, non-fatal myocardial infarction, and stroke. Further research is needed to examine effect of pharmacological approaches for the management of hyperglycemia on CVD.

Diabetic vasculopathy can be improved by *lowering blood pressure* with antihypertensive drugs which have antiatherogenic effects, e.g., ACE inhibitors, angiotensin II receptor blockers, beta-blockers, and calcium channel blockers. Randomized controlled trials like UKPDS [33, 127], HOT (Hypertension Optimal Treatment) [156], SHEP (the Systolic Hypertension in the Elderly Program) [157–159], Syst-EUR (Systolic Hypertension in Europe) [158–161], HOPE (Heart Outcomes Prevention Evaluation) [162], LIFE (Losartan Intervention For Endpoint Reduction in Hypertension) [163], and ALLHAT (the Anti-hypertensive and Lipid-Lowering Treatment to Prevent Heart Attack Trial) [164] have found beneficial effects of adequately controlling blood pressure in improving CV outcomes, specifically, for stroke, when aggressive blood pressure targets are met [33, 156, 165, 166].

Dyslipidemia plays a significant role in CV complications in T2DM. Dyslipidemia comprises elevated total cholesterol and LDL cholesterol, decreased HDL cholesterol, and high triglyceride levels [74, 75]. Lowering LDL cholesterol reduces the risk of major vascular events in T2DM patients [167]. Randomized clinical trials in T2DM have consistently shown that statins significantly reduce the risk of major primary and secondary CVD endpoints. Clinical trials of fibrate therapy have shown mixed results.

Clinical trials e.g. CARDS (the Collaborative Atorvastatin Diabetes Study) [168], LIPID (Long-term Intervention with Pravastatin in Ischemic Disease) [169], 4S (Scandinavian Simvastatin Survival Study) [170] and HPS (the Heart Protection Study) [171], demonstrated that statin significantly reduced the incidence of stroke in diabetic patients.

Subgroup analysis of the Helsinki Heart Study [136], and VA-HIT (Veterans Affairs High-density lipoprotein Intervention Trial) [172, 173] provided evidence for the potential benefit of fibrate therapy in reducing CVD in T2DM. However, FIELD (Fenofibrate Intervention and Event Lowering in Diabetes) study [174] failed to show similar benefits. The lipid arm of the ACCORD study examined combination therapy of statin and fibrate and failed to support the effectiveness to reduce CV risk as compared with statin alone [175].

Antiplatelet drugs reduce the risk of CV events in T2DM patients. Currently, aspirin is widely recommended for primary prevention of CV events in T2DM patients and is the main drug under investigation to reduce the risk of CVD [176]. Aspirin reduces the risk of serious vascular events in high risk patients by about 25% and also prevents the recurrence of angina, heart attack and stroke. Aspirin is routinely given for primary prevention of CV events in T2DM patients as all major guidelines recommend such preventive use that is based on evidence gathered from clinical trials of high-risk patients [177, 178]. However, the POPADAD (Prevention of Progression of Arterial Disease and Diabetes) trial [179] demonstrated that aspirin failed to prevent a first CV event or death in T2DM patients, which contradicts the recommendations by many guidelines. The POPADAD trial recommended that aspirin should be used for secondary prevention of CVD in patients with T2DM. The JPAD (Japanese Primary Prevention of Atherosclerosis with Aspirin for Diabetes) trial examined the efficacy of low-dose aspirin for the primary prevention of atherosclerotic events in T2DM patients and found that low-dose aspirin when used for primary prevention did not reduce the risk of CV events [180].

In a subgroup analysis of the CAPRIE (Clopidogrel versus Aspirin in Patients at Risk of Ischaemic Events) study, patients with T2DM taking clopidogrel seem to derive enhanced benefit from clopidogrel compared with aspirin [181, 182]. The subgroup analysis of PRISMPLUS (Platelet Inhibition in Ischemic Syndrome Management in Patients Limited by Unstable Signs and Symptoms) trial showed that triple therapy (aspirin, heparin, tirofiban) significantly reduced the incidence of myocardial infarction or death as compared with aspirin plus heparin [183].

9. Conclusion and recommendations

CV complications are the major causes of morbidity and mortality in patients with T2DM. Macrovascular complications are more common, and most diabetic patients develop or die of macrovascular diseases, predominantly by developing CVD.

The initiators of vasculopathy that ultimately develop into long-term complications can be controlled and avoided by strict glycemic control, maintaining normal lipid profiles, regular physical exercise, adopting a healthy lifestyle and pharmacological interventions. Studies have shown that lifestyle interventions help in prevention and reduction of CV risk factors; however, there is a lack of studies investigating effects of lifestyle modifications on long-term CV outcomes that need to be addressed. Similarly, because the intensive glycemic control in T2DM patients did not show consistent beneficial effects on CV events, such a strict glycemic control needs to be revisited. Contrary to the disappointing results of intensive glucose control in prevention of CVD, intensive control of blood pressure using anti-hypertensive drugs, normalization of lipid profiles using lipid-lowering agents, and prevention of atherosclerosis and vascular thrombosis with antiplatelet therapy have been found to be beneficial.

Health promotion and patient education should be given priority to combat CV complications in T2DM patients. A multidisciplinary approach involving patients, health professionals, and researchers should be undertaken to reduce the incidence and prevalence of T2DM and CVD, and improve the quality of life and well-being of patients.

Author details

Sayeeda Rahman[1], Md. Anwarul Azim Majumder[2*], Russell Kabir[3], Mainul Haque[4], Subir Gupta[2], Sana Mohammad Yasir Arafat[5], Nkemcho Ojeh[2] and Prasad Dalvi[6]

*Address all correspondence to: azim.majumder@cavehill.uwi.edu

1 Department of Clinical Sciences, Faculty of Life Sciences, School of Medical Sciences, University of Bradford, UK

2 Faculty of Medical Sciences, The University of the West Indies, Cave Hill Campus, Barbados, West Indies

3 Department for Allied and Public Health, Faculty of Medical Sciences, Anglia Ruskin University, Chelmsford, Essex, UK

4 Faculty of Medicine and Defense Health, National Defense University of Malaysia, Kuala Lumpur, Malaysia

5 Department of Psychiatry, Bangabandhu Sheikh Mujib Medical University, Dhaka, Bangladesh

6 Lake Erie College of Osteopathic Medicine, Bradenton, Florida, USA

References

[1] Stemmer EA. Diabetes mellitus and vascular disease. In: Aronow WS, Stemmer EA, Wilson SE, editors. Vascular Disease in the Elderly. Armonk: Futura; 1997. pp. 199-220

[2] Ness J, Nassimiha D, Feria MI, Aronow WS. Diabetes mellitus in older African-Americans, Hispanics, and whites in an academic hospital-based geriatrics practice. Coronary Artery Disease. 1999;**10**:343-346

[3] IDF. Diabetes Atlas. Brussels: International Diabetes Federation; 2003

[4] UKPDS Group. UK Prospective Diabetes Study 17: A nine-year update of a randomized, controlled trial on the effect of improved metabolic control on complications in non-insulin-dependent diabetes mellitus. Annals of Internal Medicine 1996;**124**:136-145

[5] Barceló A, Aedo C, Rajpathak S, Robles S. The cost of diabetes in Latin America and the Caribbean. Bulletin of the World Health Organization. 2003;**81**:19-27

[6] Arredondo A, Zúñiga A. Economic consequences of epidemiological changes in diabetes in middle-income countries. Diabetes Care 2004;**27**:104-109

[7] Ooyub S, Ismail F, Daud NA. Diabetes program in Malaysia – Current and future. NCD Malaysia. 2004;**3**:6-12

[8] Garcia MJ, McNamara PM, Gordon T, Kannell WB. Morbidity and mortality in diabetics in the Framingham population. Sixteen year follow-up study. Diabetes. 1974;**23**:105-111

[9] Stamler J, Vaccaro O, Neaton JD, Wentworth D. Diabetes, other risk factors, and 12-yr cardiovascular mortality for men screened in the Multiple Risk Factor Intervention Trial. Diabetes Care. 1993;**16**:434-444

[10] American Diabetes Association. Management of dyslipidemia in adults with diabetes. American Diabetes Association: Clinical Practice Recommendations 1999. Diabetes Care. 1999;**22**:556-559

[11] Rahman S, Ismail AA, Ismail SB, Naing NN, Rahman AR. Early manifestation of macrovasculopathy in newly diagnosed never treated type II diabetic patients with no traditional CVD risk factors. Diabetes Research and Clinical Practice. 2008;**80**:253-258. DOI: 10.1016/j.diabres.2007.12.2010

[12] Giannattasio C, Failla M, Capra A, et al. Increased arterial stiffness in normoglycemic normotensive offspring of type 2 diabetic parents. Hypertension. 2008;**51**:182-187. DOI: 10.1161/HYPERTENSIONAHA.107.097535

[13] Rahman S, Ismail AA, Ismail SB, Naing NN, Rahman AR. Increased arterial stiffness in normoglycaemic offspring of newly diagnosed, never treated type 2 diabetic and impaired glucose tolerance parents. The British Journal of Diabetes & Vascular Disease. 2009;**9**:65-68

[14] World Health Organisation. Diabetes. 2017. Available from: http://www.who.int/mediacentre/factsheets/fs312/en/index.html [Accessed: 11-03-2017]

[15] International Diabetes Federation. IDF Diabetes Atlas 2015. 7th ed. Brussels: IDF, 2015

[16] World Health Organization. Cardiovascular Diseases. 2017. Available from: http://www.who.int/cardiovascular_diseases/en/ [Accessed: 11-30-2017]

[17] Li H, Oldenburg B, Chamberlain C, O'Neil A, Xue B, Jolley D, Hall R, Dong Z, Guo Y. Diabetes prevalence and determinants in adults in China mainland from 2000 to 2010: A systematic review. Diabetes Research and Clinical Practice. 2012 Nov;**98**(2):226-235

[18] Rahman S, Rahman T, Ismail AA, Rashid AR. Diabetes-associated macrovasculopathy: Pathophysiology and pathogenesis. Diabetes, Obesity & Metabolism 2007;**9**:767-780

[19] Virsaladze D, Kipiani V. Endothelial dysfunction in diabetic vasculopathy. Annals of Biochemical Research and Education. 2001;**1**:44-48

[20] Cooper ME, Bonnet F, Oldfield M, Jandeleit-Dahm K. Mechanisms of diabetic vasculopathy: An overview. American Journal of Hypertension. 2001;**14**:475-486

[21] Clark CM Jr, Lee DA. Prevention and treatment of the complications of diabetes mellitus. New England Journal of Medicine. 1995;**332**:1210-1217

[22] Rahman S, Majumder MAA. Diabetes and macrovasculopthy: Double trouble. South East Asia Journal of Public Health. 2013:**3**(2):1-3

[23] Haffner SM, Alexander CM, Cook TJ, et al. Reduced coronary events in simvastatin-treated patients with coronary heart disease and diabetes or impaired fasting glucose levels: Subgroup analyses in the Scandinavian Simvastatin Survival Study. Archives of Internal Medicine. 1999;**159**:2661-2667

[24] Rahman S, Majumder MAA. Links between Vitamin D deficiency and macrovascular diseases. South East Asia Journal of Public Health. 2015:**5**(2):3-6

[25] Sowers JR. Diabetes mellitus and cardiovascular disease in women. Archives of Internal Medicine. 1998;**158**:617-621

[26] Singer DE, Moulton AW, Nathan, DM. Diabetic myocardial infarction: Interaction of diabetes with other preinfarction risk factors. Diabetes. 1989;**38**:350-357

[27] Smith JW, Marcus FI, Serokman R. Prognosis of patients with diabetes mellitus after acute myocardial infarction. American Journal of Cardiology. 1984;**54**:718-721

[28] Nathan DM, Cleary PA, Backlund JY, et al. Intensive diabetes treatment and cardiovascular disease in patients with type 1 diabetes. New England Journal of Medicine. 2005;**353**:2643-2653

[29] Wingard DL, Barrett-Connor EL, Scheidt-Nave C et al. Prevalence of cardiovascular and renal complications in older adults with normal or impaired glucose tolerance or NIDDM: a population-based study. Diabetes Care. 1993;**16**:1022-1025

[30] UK Prospective Diabetes Study 6. Complications in newly diagnosed type 2 diabetic patients and their association with different clinical and biochemical risk factors. Diabetes Research. 1990 Jan;**13**(1):1-11

[31] Balkau B, Pyörälä M, Shipley M, Forhan A, Jarrett J, Eschwège E, Pyörälä K. Non-cardiovascular disease mortality and diabetes mellitus. Lancet. 1997;**350**:1680

[32] King's Fund. Counting the Cost. The Real Impact of Non-Insulin Dependent Diabetes. British Diabetic Association; London. 1996

[33] UKPDS Group. Tight blood pressure control and risk of macrovascular and microvascular complications in type 2 diabetes (UKPDS 38). BMJ. 1998;**317**:703-713

[34] Siitonen OI, Niskanen LK, Laakso M et al. Lower-extremity amputations in diabetic and non-diabetic patients. Diabetes Care. 1993;**16**:16

[35] Beckman JA, Creager MA, Libby P. Diabetes and atherosclerosis. JAMA. 2002;**287**: 2570-2581

[36] Seligman BG, Biolo A, Polanczyk CA, Gross JL, Clausell N. Increased plasma levels of endothelin 1 and van Willbrand factor in patients with type 2 diabetic mellitus and dyslipidaemia. Diabetes Care. 2000;**23**:1395-1400

[37] Luscher TF, Creager MA, Beckman JA, Cosentino F. Diabetes and vascular disease: Pathophysiology, clinical consequences and medical therapy: Part II. Circulation. 2003;**108**:1655-1661

[38] Creager MA, Luscher TF, Cosentino F, Beckman JA. Diabetes and vascular disease: Pathophysiology, clinical consequences and medical therapy: Part I. Circulation. 2003;**108**:1527-1532

[39] Beckman JA. Pathophysiology of vascular dysfunction in diabetes. Cardiology Rounds. 2004;**8**

[40] Kadirvelu A, Han CK, Lang CC. Endothelial dysfunction in cardiovascular diseases. Medical Progress. 2002;**5**:4-10

[41] Taylor PD, Poston L. The effect of hyperglycaemia on function of rat isolated mesenteric resistance artery. British Journal of Pharmacology. 1994;**113**:801-808

[42] Tooke JE. Microvascular function in human diabetes. Diabetes. 1995;**44**:721-726

[43] Rattan V, Sultana C, Shen Y, Kaba VK. Oxidant stress induced trans endothelial migration of monocytes is linked to phosphorylation of PECAM-1. American Journal of Physiology. 1997;**273**:E453-E461

[44] Tesfamariam B, Brown ML, Cohen RA. Elevated glucose impaired endothelium-dependent relaxation by activating protein kinase C. Journal of Clinical Investigation. 1991;**87**:1643-1648

[45] Paston L, Taylor PD. Endothelium-mediated vascular function in insulin-dependent diabetes mellitus. Circulation Research. 1995;**88**:245-255

[46] Ruderman NB, Haudenschild C. Diabetes as an atherogenic factor. Progress in Cardiovascular Diseases. 1984;**26**:373-412

[47] Fukumoto H, Naito Z, Asano G, Aramaki T. Immunohistochemical and morphometric evaluations of coronary atherosclerotic plaques associated with myocardial infarction and diabetes mellitus. Journal of Atherosclerosis and Thrombosis. 1998;**5**:29-35

[48] Walsh MF, Dominguez LJ, Sowers JR. Metabolic abnormalities in cardiac ischemia. Cardiology Clinics. 1995;**13**:529-538

[49] Stein B, Weintraub WS, Gebhart S. Influence of diabetes mellitus on early and late outcome after percutaneous transluminal coronary angioplasty. Circulation. 1995:**91**:979-989

[50] Winocour PD, Bryszewska M, Watula C. Reduced membrane fluidity in platelets from diabetic patients. Diabetes. 1990;**39**:241-244

[51] Davi G, Catalons I, Averna M. Thromboxane biosynthesis and platelet function in type II diabetes mellitus. New England Journal of Medicine. 1990;**322**:1768-1774

[52] Vlassara H. Recent progress in advanced glycation end products and diabetic complications. Diabetes. 1997;**46**(Suppl. 2):S19-S25

[53] Parving HH, Nielsen FS, Bang LE et al. Macromicroangiopathy and endothelium dysfunction in NIDDM patients with and without diabetic nephropathy. Diabetologia. 1996;**39**:1590-1597

[54] Chaturvedi N, Fuller JH, Pokras F, Rottiers R, Papazoglou N, Aiello LP. Circulating plasma vascular endothelial growth factor and microvascular complications of type I diabetes mellitus: The influence of ACE inhibition. Diabetic Medicine. 2001;**18**:288-294

[55] García Frade LJ, de la Calle H, Alava I, Navarro JL, Creight LJ, Gaffney LJ. Diabetes mellitus as an hypercoagulable state: Its relationship with fibrin fragments and vascular damage. Thrombosis Research. 1987;**47**:533-540

[56] Ford I, Singh TP, Kitchen S, Makris M, Ward JD, Preston FE. Activation of coagulation in diabetes mellitus in relation to the presence of vascular complications. Diabetic Medicine. 1991;**8**:322-329

[57] Carmassi F, Morale M, Puccetti R. Coagulation and fibrinolytic system impairment in insulin dependent diabetes mellitus. Thrombosis Research. 1992;**67**:643-654

[58] Sowers JR, Tuck ML, Sowers DK. Plasma antithrombin III and thrombin generation time: Correlation with hemoglobin A1 and fasting serum glucose in young diabetic women. Diabetes Care. 1980;**3**:655-658

[59] Ramirez LC, Arauz-Pacheco C, Lackner C. Lipoprotein (a) levels in diabetes mellitus: Relationship to metabolic control. Annals of Internal Medicine. 1992;**117**:42-47

[60] Ceriello A, Quatraro A, Dello Russo P. Protein C deficiency in insulin dependent diabetes: A hyperglycemia related phenomenon. Thrombosis & Haemostasis. 1990;**64**:104-107

[61] Vukovich TC, Proidl S, Knobl P, Teufelsbauer H, Schnack C, Schernthaner G. The effect of insulin treatment on the balance between tissue plasminogen activator and plasminogen activator inhibitor-1 in type 2 diabetic patients. Thrombosis & Haemostasis. 1992;**68**:253-256

[62] Laakso M. Hyperglycaemia and cardiovascular disease in type 2 diabetes. Diabetes. 1999;**48**:937-942

[63] Grundy SM, Benjamin IJ, Burke GL et al. Diabetes and cardiovascular disease: A statement for healthcare professionals from the American Heart Association. Circulation. 1999;**100**:1134-1146

[64] The Diabetes Control and Complications Trial Research Group. The effect of intensive treatment of diabetes on the development and progression of long term complications in insulin-dependent diabetes mellitus. New England Journal of Medicine. 1993;**329**:977-986

[65] Bayes JW. Role of oxidative stress in development of complications in diabetes. Diabetes. 1991;**40**:405-412

[66] Morigi M, Angioletti S, Imberti B et al. Leukocyte endothelial interaction is augmented by high glucose concentrations and hyperglycemia in a NF-kB-dependent fashion. Journal of Clinical Investigation. 1998;**101**:1905-1915

[67] Sowers JR, Epstein M. Risk factors for arterial disease in diabetes: Hypertension. In: Tooke JE, editor. Diabetic Angiopathy. London: Arnold Publishers;1999:45-63

[68] Tribe RM, Poston L. Oxidative stress and lipids in diabetes: A role in endothelial vasodilator function? Vascular Medicine. 1996;**1**:195-206

[69] McMillen DE. Development of vascular complications in diabetes. Vascular Medicine. 1997;**2**:132-142

[70] Baumgartner-Parzer SM, Wagner L, Pettermann M, Gessel A, Waldhiäusi W. Modulation by high glucose of adhesion molecule expression in cultured endothelial cells. Diabetologia. 1995;**38**:1367-1370

[71] King GL, Brownlee M. The cellular and molecular mechanisms of diabetic complications. Endocrinology and Metabolism Clinics of North America. 1996;**25**:255-270

[72] Cooper ME, Cao Z, Rumble JR, Jandeleit K, Allen TJ, Gilbert RE. Attenuation of diabetes-associated mesenteric vascular hypertrophy with perindopril: Morphological and molecular biological studies. Metabolism. 1998;**47**:24-27

[73] Aronson D, Rayfield EJ. How hyperglycemia promotes atherosclerosis: Molecular mechanisms. Cardiovascular Diabetology. 2002;**1**:1

[74] Watkins PJ. ABC of diabetes cardiovascular disease, hypertension, and lipids. BMJ. 2003; **326**:874-886

[75] Georg P, Ludvik B. Lipids and diabetes. Journal of Clinical and Basic Cardiology. 2000; 3:159-162

[76] Steinberg D. Low density lipoprotein oxidation and its pathobiological significance. Journal of Biological Chemistry. 1997;**272**:20963-20966

[77] Khoo JC, Miller E, McLoughlin P, Steinberg D. Enhanced macrophage uptake of low-density lipoprotein after self-aggregation. Atherosclerosis. 1988;**8**:348-358

[78] Ross R. Atherosclerosis – An inflammatory disease. New England Journal of Medicine. 1999;**340**:115-126

[79] Ferri C, Bellini C, Desideri G et al. Plasma endothelin-1 in obese hypertensive and normotensive man. Diabetes. 1995;**44**:431-436

[80] Hunter SJ, Garvey T. Insulin action and insulin resistance: Diseases involving defects in insulin receptors, signal transduction and glucose transport effector system. American Journal of Medicine. 1998;**5**:331-346

[81] Sowers JR, Sowers PS, Peuler JD. Role of insulin resistance and hyper-insulinemia in development of hypertension and atherosclerosis. Journal of Laboratory and Clinical Medicine. 1994;**123**:647-652

[82] Reaven GM, Lithell H, Landsberg L. Hypertension and associated metabolic abnormalities: The role of insulin resistance and sympathetic adrenal system. New England Journal of Medicine. 1996;**334**:374-381

[83] Gilbert RE, Rumble JR, Cao ZM et al. Endothelin receptor antagonism ameliorates mast cell infiltration, vascular hypertrophy, and epidermal growth factor expression in experimental diabetes. Circulation Research. 2000;**86**:158-165

[84] Myllärniemi M, Calderon L, Lemström K, Buchdunger E, Häyry P. Inhibition of platelet-derived growth factors receptor kinase inhibits smooth muscle cell migration and proliferation. FASEB Journal. 1997;**11**:1111-1126

[85] Feener EP, King GL. Vascular dysfunction in diabetes mellitus. Lancet. 1997;**350**(Suppl. 1): S9-S13

[86] Koya D, King GL. Protein kinase C activation and the development of diabetic complications. Diabetes. 1998;**47**:859-866

[87] Storey AM, Perry CJ, Petrie JR. Endothelial dysfunction in type 2 diabetes. The British Journal of Diabetes & Vascular Disease. 2001;**1**:22-27

[88] Brodsky S, Chen J, Lee A, Akassoglou K, Norman J, Goligorsky MS. Plasmin dependent and independent effects of plasminogen activators and inhibitor-1 on ex-vivo angiogenesis. American Journal of Physiology. 2001;**281**:H1784-H1792

[89] Nishikawa T, Edelstein D, Du XL et al. Normalizing mitochondrial superoxide production blocks three pathways of hyperglycaemic damage. Nature. 2000;**404**:787-790

[90] Baynes JW, Thorpe SR. Role of oxidative stress in diabetic complications: A new perspective on an old paradigm. Diabetes. 1999;**48**:1-9

[91] Baynes JW. Role of oxidative stress in development of complications in diabetes. Diabetes. 1991;**40**:405-412

[92] Vozarova B, Weyer C, Lindsay RS, Pratley RE, Bogardus C, Tataranni PA. High WBC count is associated with a worsening of insulin sensitivity and predicts the development of type 2 diabetes. Diabetes. 2002;**51**:455-461

[93] Tuttle HA, Davis-Gorman G, Goldman S, Copeland JG, McDonagh PF. Platelet neutrophil conjugate formation is increased in diabetic women with cardiovascular disease. Cardiovascular Diabetology. 2003;**2**:1-16

[94] Sower JR, Lester MA. Diabetes and cardiovascular disease. Diabetes Care. 1998;**22**(Suppl. 3): c.14-c.20

[95] Ernst E, Hammerschmidt DE, Bagge U, Matrai A, Dormandy JA. Leukocytes and the risk of ischemic diseases. JAMA. 1987;**257**:2318-2324

[96] Fusman R, Rotstein R, Zeltser D et al. The state of leukocyte adhesiveness/aggregation in the peripheral blood of patients with type 2 diabetes and ischemic vascular disease. Acta Diabetologica. 2001;**38**:43-49

[97] Benetos A, Weaber B, Izzo J, Mitchell G, Resnick L, et al. Influence of age, risk factors, and cardiovascular and renal disease on arterial stiffness: Clinical application. American Journal of Hypertension. 2002;**15**:1101-1108

[98] Safar ME, London GM. The arterial system in human hypertension. In: Swales JD editor., Textbook of Hypertension. London: Blackwell Scientific; 1994

[99] Asmar R, Benetos A, Topouchian J, Laurent, P, et al. Assessment of arterial distensibility by automatic pulse wave velocity measurement. Validation and clinical application studies. Hypertension. 1995;**26**:85-490

[100] Tanaka H, DeSouza CA, Seals DR. Absence of age-related increase in central artery stiffness in physically active women. Arteriosclerosis, Thrombosis, and Vascular Biology. 1998. **18**:127-132

[101] Westerbacka J, Vehkavaara S, Bergholm R, et al. Marked resistance of the ability of insulin to decrease arterial stiffness characterizes human obesity. Diabetes. 1999;**48**:821-827

[102] Westerbacka J, Wilkinson I, Cockcroft J, et al. Diminished wave reflection in the aorta: A novel physiological action of insulin on large blood vessels. Hypertension. 1999;**33**:1118-1122

[103] Wilkinson IB, Cockcroft JR, Webb DJ. Pulse wave analysis and arterial stiffness. Journal of Cardiovascular Pharmacology. 1999;**32**:33-37

[104] O'Rourke MF, Hayward CS. Arterial stiffness, gender and heart rate. Journal of Hypertension. 2003;**21**:487-490

[105] Mackenzie IS, Wilkinson IB, Cockcroft JR. Assessment of arterial stiffness in clinical practice. Quarterly Journal of Medicine. 2002;**95**:67-74

[106] Safar ME, Henry O, Meaume S. Aortic pulse wave velocity: An independent marker of cardiovascular risk. The American Journal of Geriatric Cardiology. 2002;**11**:295-298

[107] O'Rourke MF, Pauca A, Jiang X. Pulse wave analysis. British Journal of Clinical Pharmacology 2001;**51**:507-522

[108] Wilkinson IB, Cockcroft JR, Webb DJ. Pulse wave analysis and arterial stiffness. Journal of Cardiovascular Pharmacology. 1998;**32**:S33-S37

[109] Wilkinson IB, Fuchs SA, Jansen IM et al. Reproducibility of pulse wave velocity and augmentation index measured by pulse wave analysis. Journal of Hypertension. 1998;**16**:2079-2084

[110] Kelly R, Hayward C, Avolio A, O'Rourke M. Noninvasive determination of age-related changes in the human arterial pulse. Circulation 1989;**80**:1652-1659

[111] Cameron JD, McGrath BP, Dart AM. Use of radial applanation tonometry and a generalized transfer function to determine aortic augmentation in subjects with treated hypertension. Journal of the American College of Cardiology 1998;**32**:1214-1220

[112] Wilkinson IB, MacCallum H, Flint L, Cockcroft JR et al. The influence of heart rate on augmentation index and central arterial pressure. Journal of Physiology 2000;**525**:263-270

[113] Wilkinson IB, Prasad K, Hall IR, Thomas A, MacCallum H. et al. Increased central pulse pressure and augmentation index in subjects with hypercholesterolemia. Journal of the American College of Cardiology. 2002;**39**:1005-1011

[114] Rehman A, Rahman ARA, Rasool AHG. Effect of angiotensin II on pulse wave velocity in humans is mediated through angiotensin II type 1 (AT_1) receptors. Journal of Human Hypertension. 2002;**16**:261-266

[115] Chowienczyk PJ, Kelly RP, MacCallum H, Millasseau SC, et al. Photoplethysmographic assessment of pulse wave reflection. Journal of the American College of Cardiology. 1999;**34**:2007-2014

[116] Resnick LM, Militianu D, Cunnings AJ, Pipe JG, et al. Direct magnetic resonance determination of aortic distensibility in essential hypertension: Relation to age, abdominal visceral fat and in situ intracellular free magnesium. Hypertension. 1997;**30**:654-659

[117] Mohiaddin RH, Underwood SR, Bogren HG, Firmin DN, et al. Regional aortic compliance studied by magnetic resonance imaging: The effects of age, training and coronary artery disease. British Heart Journal. 1989:**62**:90-96

[118] Rahman S, Majumder MAA, Rahman ARA. Treatment of diabetic vasculopathy: An overview. Research and Reports in Endocrine Disorders. 2011;**1**:21-36

[119] Emoto M, Nishizawa Y, Kawagishi T, Maekawa K, Hiura Y, et al. Stiffness indexes ß of the common carotid and femoral arteries are associated with insulin resistance in NIDDM. Diabetes Care. 1998;**21**:1178-1182

[120] Ngim CA, Rahman ARA, Ibrahim A. Pulse wave velocity as an index of arterial stiffness: A comparison between newly diagnosed (untreated) hypertensive and normotensive middle-aged Malay men and its relationship with fasting insulin. Acta Cardiologica. 1999;**54**:277-282

[121] Rahman S, Ismail AA, Rahman AR. Treatment of diabetic vasculopathy with rosiglitazone and ramipril: Hype or hope? International Journal of Diabetes in Developing Countries. 2009;**29**:110-117

[122] American Diabetes Association. Position statement: Diabetes mellitus and exercise. Diabetes Care. 1990;**13**:804-805

[123] Dela F, Ploug T, Handberg A, et al. Physical training increases muscle GLUT 4 protein and mRNA in patients with NIDDM. Diabetes. 1994;**7**:862-865

[124] Lebovitz HE, Feinglos MN. Mechanism of action of the second generation sulfonylurea glipizide. American Journal of Medicine. 1983;**75**:46-54

[125] Kolterman OG, Gra RS, Shapiro G, Scarlett JA, Griffin J, Olesfsky JM. The acute and chronic effects of sulfonylurea therapy in type II diabetic subjects. Diabetes. 1984;**33**:346-354

[126] Groop L. Metabolic effects of sulfonylurea drugs. A review. Ann Clin Res. 1983;**15**(Suppl 37):16-20

[127] Hanefeld M, Schaper F. The role of alpha-glucosidase inhibitors (Acarbose). In: Mogensen CE, editor. Pharmacotherapy of Diabetes: New Developments. Improving Life and Prognosis for Diabetic Patients. New York, NY: Springer; 2007. pp. 143-152

[128] McDougall C, McKay GA, Fisher M. Drugs for diabetes: Part 6 GLP-1receptor agonists. British Journal of Cardiology. 2011;**18**:167-169

[129] McDougall C, McKay GA, Fisher M. Drugs for diabetes: Part 5 DPP-4 inhibitors. British Journal of Cardiology. 2011;**18**:130-132

[130] Nauck M, Smith U. Incretin-based therapy: How do incretin mimetics and DPP-4 inhibitors fit into treatment algorithms for type 2 diabetic patients? Best Practice & Research. Clinical Endocrinology & Metabolism. 2009;**23**:513-523

[131] Siddiqui NI. Incretinmimetics and DPP-4 inhibitors: New approach to treatment of type 2 diabetes mellitus. Mymensingh Medical Journal. 2009;**18**(1):113-124

[132] Joint National Committee on Prevention, Detection, Evaluation, and Treatment of High Blood Pressure. The Seventh Report of the Joint National Committee on Prevention, Detection, Evaluation and Treatment of High Blood Pressure. Bethesda, MD: National Heart, Lung, and Blood Institute (US); 2004

[133] McFarlane SI, Kumar A, Sowers JR. Mechanisms by which angiotensin converting enzyme inhibitors prevent diabetes and cardiovascular disease. American Journal of Cardiology. 2003;**91**(12A):30H-37H

[134] Mayor S. Calcium channel blockers associated with less diabetes. BMJ. 2006;**333**:514

[135] Pyörälä K, Pedersen TR, Kjekshus J, Faergeman O, Olsson AG, Thorgeirsson G. Cholesterol lowering with simvastatin improves Prognosis of diabetic patients with coronary heart disease. A subgroup analysis of the Scandinavian Simvastatin Survival Study (4S). Diabetes Care. 1997;**20**:614-620

[136] Koskinen P, Manttari M, Manninen V, Huttunen JK, Heinonen OP, Frick MH. Coronary heart disease incidence in NIDDM patients in the Helsinki Heart Study. Diabetes Care. 1992;**15**:820-825

[137] Zanchetti A. Aspirin and antiplatelet drugs in the prevention of cardiovascular complications of diabetes. In: Mogensen CE, editor. Pharmacotherapy of Diabetes: New Developments. Improving Life and Prognosis for Diabetic Patients. New York, NY: Springer; 2007. pp. 211-218

[138] Sacks FM, Pfeffer MA, Moye LA, et al. The effect of pravastatin on coronary events after myocardial infarction in patients with average cholesterol levels. Cholesterol

and Recurrent Events Trial investigators. New England Journal of Medicine. 1996;**335**: 1001-1009

[139] The Long-term Intervention with Pravastatin in Ischaemic Disease (LIPID) Study Group. Prevention of cardiovascular events and death with pravastatin in patients with coronary heart disease and a broad range of initial cholesterol levels. New England Journal of Medicine. 1998;**339**:1349-1357

[140] Elkeles RS, Diamond JR, Poulter C, et al. Cardiovascular outcomes in type 2 diabetes. A double-blind placebo-controlled study of bezafibrate: The St Mary's, Ealing, Northwick Park Diabetes Cardiovascular Disease Prevention (SENDCAP) Study. Diabetes Care. 1998;**21**:641-648

[141] Rubins HB, Robins SJ, Collins D, et al. Gemfibrozil for the secondary prevention of coronary heart disease in men with low levels of high density lipoprotein cholesterol. New England Journal of Medicine. 1999;**341**:410-418

[142] Diabetes Atherosclerosis Intervention Study Investigators. Effect of fenofibrate on progression of coronary-artery disease in type 2 diabetes: The Diabetes Atherosclerosis Intervention Study, a randomised study. Lancet. 2001;**357**:905-910

[143] Hankey GJ, Eikelboom JW. Antiplatelet drugs. Medical Journal of Australia. 2003;**178**: 568-574

[144] Gillies CL, Abrams KR, Lambert PC, et al. Pharmacological and lifestyle interventions to prevent or delay type 2 diabetes in people with impaired glucose tolerance: Systematic review and meta-analysis. BMJ. 2007;**334**:299

[145] Stiegler RS, Zimmet PZ, Cameron AJ, et al. Lifestyle management: Preventing type 2 diabetes and cardiovascular complications. Therapy. 2009;**6**:489-496

[146] UK Prospective Diabetes Study (UKPDS) Group. Effect of intensive blood-glucose control with metformin on complications in overweight patients with type 2 diabetes (UKPDS 34). Lancet. 1998;**352**:854-865

[147] Patel A, MacMahon S, Chalmers J, et al. Intensive blood glucose control and vascular outcomes in patients with Type 2 diabetes. New England Journal of Medicine. 2008;**358**:2560-2572

[148] Schor S. The University Group Diabetes Program. A statistician looks at the mortality results. JAMA. 1971;**217**:1671-1675

[149] Action to Control Cardiovascular Risk in Diabetes Study Group. Effects of intensive glucose lowering in type 2 diabetes. New England Journal of Medicine. 2008;**358**:2545-2559

[150] UK Prospective Diabetes Study (UKPDS) Group. Intensive blood-glucose control with sulphonylureas or insulin compared with conventional treatment and risk of complications in patients with type 2 diabetes (UKPDS 33). Lancet. 1998;**352**:837-853

[151] Shichiri M, Kishikawa H, Ohkubo Y, Wake N. Long-term results of the Kumamoto Study on optimal diabetes control in type 2 diabetic patients. Diabetes Care. 2000;**23** Suppl 2:B21-B29

[152] Holman RR, Paul SK, Bethel MA, Matthews DR, Neil HA. 10-year follow-up of intensive glucose control in type 2 diabetes. New England Journal of Medicine 2008;**359**:1577-1589

[153] Duckworth W, Abraira C, Moritz T, et al. VADT Investigators. Glucose control and vascular complications in veterans with type 2 diabetes. New England Journal of Medicine. 2009;**360**:129-139

[154] Nathan DM. Navigating the choices for diabetes prevention. New England Journal of Medicine 2010;**362**:1533-1535

[155] Dormandy JA, Charbonnel B, Eckland DJ, et al. PROactive investigators. Secondary prevention of macrovascular events in patients with type 2 diabetes in the PROactive Study (PROspectivepioglitAzone Clinical Trial In macroVascular Events): A randomised controlled trial. Lancet. 2005;**366**:1279-1289

[156] Hansson L, Zanchetti A, Carruthers SG, et al. Effects of intensive blood pressure lowering and low-dose aspirin in patients with hypertension: Principal results of the Hypertension Optimal Treatment (HOT) randomised trial. HOT Study Group. Lancet. 1998;**351**:1755-1762

[157] SHEP Cooperative Research Group. Prevention of stroke by Antihypertensive drug treatment in older persons with isolated systolic hypertension. Final results of the Systolic Hypertension in the Elderly Program (SHEP). JAMA. 1991;**265**:3255-3264

[158] Staessen JA, Fagard R, Thijs L, et al. Randomised double-blind comparison of placebo and active treatment for older patients with isolated systolic hypertension. The Systolic Hypertension in Europe (Syst-Eur) Trial Investigators. Lancet. 1997;**350**:757-764

[159] Staessen JA, Thijs L, Gasowski J, Cells H, Fagard RH. Treatment of isolated systolic hypertension in the elderly: Further evidence from the systolic hypertension in Europe (Syst-Eur) trial. American Journal of Cardiology. 1998;**82**(9B):20R-22R

[160] International Diabetes Federation (IDF). Diabetes Atlas. 4th ed. Brussels: International Diabetes Federation; 2009

[161] Voyaki SM, Staessen JA, Thijs L, et al. Follow-up of renal function in treated and untreated older patients with isolated systolic hypertension. Systolic Hypertension in Europe (Syst-Eur) Trial Investigators. Journal of Hypertension. 2001;**19**:511-519

[162] Heart Outcomes Prevention Evaluation (HOPE) Study Investigators. Effects of ramipril on cardiovascular and microvascular outcomes in people with diabetes mellitus: Results of the HOPE study and MICROHOPE substudy. Lancet. 2000;**355**:253-259

[163] Dahlöf B, Devereux RB, Kjeldsen SE, et al. Cardiovascular morbidity and mortality in the Losartan Intervention For Endpoint reduction in hypertension study (LIFE): A randomised trial against atenolol. Lancet. 2002;**359**:995-1003

[164] ALLHAT Officers and Coordinators for the ALLHAT Collaborative Research Group. Major outcomes in high-risk hypertensive patients randomized to angiotensin-converting enzyme inhibitor or calcium channel blocker vs diuretic: The Antihypertensive and Lipid-Lowering Treatment to Prevent Heart Attack Trial (ALLHAT). JAMA. 2002;**288**:2981-2997

[165] Chobanian AV, Bakris GL, Black HR, et al. The seventh Report of the Joint National Committee on Prevention, Detection, Evaluation, and Treatment of High Blood Pressure: The JNC 7 report. JAMA. 2003;**289**:2560-2572

[166] Adler AI, Stratton IM, Neil HA, et al. Association of systolic blood pressure with macrovascular and microvascular complications of type 2 diabetes (UKPDS 36): Prospective observational study. BMJ. 2000;**321**:412-419

[167] Heart Protection Study Collaborative Group. MRC/BHF Heart Protection Study of cholesterol lowering with simvastatin in 20,536 high-risk individuals: A randomised placebo-controlled trial. Lancet. 2002;**360**:7-22

[168] Colhoun HM, Betteridge DJ, Durrington PN, et al. CARDS investigators. Primary prevention of cardiovascular disease with atorvastatin in type 2 diabetes in the Collaborative Atorvastatin Diabetes Study (CARDS): Multicentre randomised placebo-controlled trial. Lancet. 2004;**364**:685-696

[169] Keech A, Colquhoun D, Best J, et al. Secondary prevention of cardiovascular events with long-term pravastatin in patients with diabetes or impaired fasting glucose: Results from the LIPID trial. Diabetes Care. 2003;**26**:2713-2721

[170] Pederson TR, Kjekshus J, Pyorala K, et al. Effect of simvastatin on ischaemic signs and symptoms in the Scandinavian simvastatin survival study (4S). American Journal of Cardiology 1998;**81**:333-335

[171] Collins R, Armitage J, Parish S, Sleigh P, Peto R. MRC/BHF Heart Protection Study of cholesterol-lowering with simvastatin in 5963 people with diabetes: A randomised placebo-controlled trial. Lancet. 2003;**361**:2005-2016

[172] Rubins HB, Robins SJ, Collins D, et al. VA-HIT Study Group. Diabetes, plasma insulin, and cardiovascular disease subgroup analysis from the Department of Veterans Affairs high-density lipoprotein intervention trial (VA-HIT). Archives of Internal Medicine. 2002;**162**:2597-2604

[173] Robins SJ, Collins D, Wittes JT, et al, VA-HIT Study Group. Veterans Affairs high-density lipoprotein intervention trial. Relation of gemfibrozil treatment and lipid levels with major coronary events: VA-HIT: A randomized controlled trial. JAMA. 2001;**285**:1585-1591

[174] Keech A, Simes RJ, Barter P, et al. Effects of long-term fenofibrate therapy on cardiovascular events in 9795 people with type 2 diabetes mellitus (the FIELD study): Randomised controlled trial. Lancet 2005;**366**:1849-1861

[175] The ACCORD Study Group. Effects of combination lipid therapy in type 2 diabetes mellitus. New England Journal of Medicine. 2010;**362**:1563-1574

[176] Pignone M, Alberts MJ, Colwell JA, et al. Aspirin for primary prevention of cardiovascular events in people with diabetes. Journal of the American College of Cardiology 2010;**55**:2878-2886

[177] Buse JB, Ginsberg HN, Bakris GL, et al, American Heart Association, American Diabetes Association. Primary prevention of cardiovascular diseases in people with diabetes mellitus: A scientific statement from the American Heart Association and the American Diabetes Association. Circulation. 2007;**115**:114-126

[178] Rydén L, Standl E, Bartnik M, et al. Guidelines on diabetes, pre-diabetes, and cardiovascular diseases: Executive summary. The Task Force on Diabetes and cardiovascular Diseases of the European Society of Cardiology (ESC) and of the European Association for the Study of Diabetes (EASD). European Heart Journal. 2007;**28**:88-136

[179] Belch J, MacCuish A, Campbell I, et al. The prevention of progression of arterial disease and diabetes (POPADAD) trial: Factorial randomised placebo controlled trial of aspirin and antioxidants in patients with diabetes and asymptomatic peripheral arterial disease. BMJ 2008;**337**:a1840

[180] Ogawa H, Nakayama M, Morimoto T, et al, Japanese Primary Prevention of Atherosclerosis With Aspirin for Diabetes (JPAD) Trial Investigators. Low-dose aspirin for primary prevention of atherosclerotic events in patients with type 2 diabetes: A randomized controlled trial. JAMA. 2008;**300**:2134-2141

[181] CAPRIE Steering Committee. A randomized, blinded trial of clopidogrel versus aspirin in patients at risk of ischemic events (CAPRIE). Lancet. 1996;**348**:1329-1339

[182] Bhatt DL, Marso SP, Hirsch AT, et al. Amplified benefit of clopidogrel versus aspirin in patients with diabetes mellitus. American Journal of Cardiology. 2002;**90**:625-628

[183] Theroux P, Alexander J Jr, Pharand C, et al. Glycoprotein IIb/IIIa receptor blockade improves outcomes in diabetic patients presenting with unstable angina/non-ST-elevation myocardial infarction: Results from the Platelet Inhibition in Ischemic Syndrome Management in Patients Limited by Unstable Signs and Symptoms (PRISM-PLUS) study. Circulation. 2001;**102**:2466-2472

Chapter 6

Iron Status Biomarkers and Cardiovascular Risk

María Pilar Vaquero, Ángel García-Quismondo,
Francisco J. del Cañizo and
Francisco J. Sánchez-Muniz

Additional information is available at the end of the chapter

http://dx.doi.org/10.5772/intechopen.69040

Abstract

Both iron excess and deficiency may be related to oxidative stress. Serum ferritin, the main marker of iron status, and hepcidin, the key regulator of iron metabolism, are increased in inflammation states and their links with insulin resistance are emerging topics. We have reviewed the role of iron deficiency/overload in cardiovascular risk, including our own results. Most studies deal with the association between iron deposition in tissues and cardiovascular risk, while decreased iron status is predominantly related to protection against atherosclerosis and coronary heart disease. Less information is available on the role of iron status in type 2 diabetes mellitus (T2DM). Serum ferritin is positively correlated with several indicators of cardiovascular risk in healthy adults and diabetics, thus excess body iron is related to cardiometabolic alterations including vascular and heart damage, central obesity, and metabolic syndrome. Our data in an ample sample of T2DM adults suggest that body iron stores, evaluated as ferritin, are clearly related with some key markers of the so-called lipidic triad (high triglyceride and low high-density lipoprotein (HDL) cholesterol) levels together with the presence of small and dense low-density lipoprotein particles which also is in the frame of the dysmetabolic iron overload syndrome.

Keywords: iron, cardiovascular diseases, iron overload, iron deficiency, oxidative stress, hepcidin, ferritin, insulin, Type 2 diabetes Mellitus, lipidic triad, biomarker, dysmetabolic iron overload syndrome, human

1. Introduction

1.1. Iron metabolism and regulation

Iron is essential for life as it plays a central role in many biological processes that involve oxygen transport and storage and oxidative metabolism. This essential metal participates in many enzymatic systems such as those involved in DNA, RNA, and protein syntheses and in the regulation of gene expression, electron transport in the mitochondria, neurotransmitter metabolism, vitamin D activation, and cholesterol catabolism through the 7α-hydroxylase linked to isoenzyme P450 cytochrome (CYP7A1c) that depends on iron and converts cholesterol to colic acid [1, 2].

Most of the functional iron in the body is present in the form of hemoglobin and myoglobin, and minor levels are part of a variety of heme and non-heme enzymes; the remainder is stored and mobilized when physiological demands are increased. The existence of two ionic forms, Fe^{2+} and Fe^{3+}, means that this nutrient is capable to serve both as an electron donor and as an acceptor, which makes iron essential but also a potential toxic. In order to limit the amount of free ions that can induce free radical formation, iron is transported, bound to proteins, and stored intracellularly within a macro-protein structure, ferritin.

Iron in food is present in two forms, inorganic iron and heme iron. These forms are absorbed by different mechanisms; the heme route is highly efficient but contributes only to about 10–15% of total dietary iron. Non-heme iron bioavailability is enhanced principally by animal tissue and ascorbic acid, whereas phytic acid and polyphenols are the main inhibitors [1, 3–6]. Solubility is an important factor for iron uptake; soluble ferrous iron is transported by the divalent metal transporter (DMT1) located at the luminal side of the duodenal membrane. However, this is not as simple; on the one hand, this carrier is not iron specific and there is competition from other divalent metals, such as calcium [7] and zinc, and on the other hand, ferric ion can be also transported either after reduction to ferrous by the duodenal cytochrome B or by interaction to mucins and subsequent association with β3-integrin and mobilferrin that cross the membrane and internalize iron in the cytosol [8, 9].

It is important to emphasize that iron absorption is tightly controlled, but once absorbed there are no excretion mechanisms. In contrast, iron recycling in the body is highly efficient; senescent erythrocytes are phagocytosed by macrophages in the liver, spleen, and bone marrow. Under normal conditions, only about 10% of the 10–18 mg/day-ingested iron is absorbed. However, during late pregnancy (from 6 to 9 months), in order to cover fetal demands for growth and erythropoiesis, iron absorption increases to 25% [10]. The main serum transporter is transferrin, a protein capable of binding 1 or 2 ferric ions that are released into cells by the transferrin receptor (TfR1). Iron recycling involves 10–20 times greater iron flux than intestinal absorption, that makes approximately 20–25 mg of iron circulating daily, an amount sufficient to ensure erythropoiesis needs. This role is played by macrophages in the spleen, bone marrow, and liver (Küpffer cells) [11]. Iron losses are due to intestinal desquamation and menstruation and should balance absorbed amounts (average 1–2 mg/day). However, hemorrhages, intense menstrual blood loss [12], pregnancy, and intense growth are frequent causes of iron deficiency anemia (IDA).

In iron overload conditions, such as hereditary hemochromatosis, transferrin becomes saturated with iron and the excess occurs as non-transferrin-bound iron (NTBI) that may be toxic [13].

The discovery of the intracellular iron regulatory proteins and that of the key regulator, hepcidin, has triggered a revolution in iron metabolism research. Hepcidin, now accepted as a true

http://dx.doi.org/10.5772/intechopen.69040

hormone, was initially named liver-expressed antimicrobial peptide (LEAP-1) and shortly later renamed as hepcidin because it is expressed in the liver (hep-) and exhibits antimicrobial activity (-cidin) [14, 15].

Figure 1 shows a scheme of the role of hepcidin on systemic iron homeostasis under conditions of high or low iron level. Hepatic hepcidin synthesis is stimulated, secreted into the circulation, and released into tissues when iron levels are high. In different cells but mainly in hepatocytes, enterocytes, and macrophages, hepcidin inhibits iron export, thus decreases absorption, recycling, and circulation of iron. This hormone therefore is a negative regulator of iron status. The mechanism of action is binding to its receptor, the cellular iron exporter ferroportin (FPN), and subsequent internalization and degradation of the hepcidin-ferroportin complex. In contrast, under physiological or pathological situations of low iron levels, hepcidin synthesis is minimized resulting in an enhanced iron flux from liver and macrophages stores and an increased transport through the duodenal basolateral membrane.

The gene-encoding hepcidin, *HAMP*, is expressed primarily in hepatocytes, although there is also evidence of expression in duodenal enterocytes, liver Kupffer cells, splenic macrophages, and placental syncytiotrophoblasts [16]. Sequencing of *HAMP* reveals several mutations that are either not functional [17] or related to a rare form of hemochromatosis [18] indicating low variability and that this gene is highly conserved in humans while the common iron metabolism alterations, either iron deficiency or hemochromatosis, have been associated with polymorphisms in other genes [19–23].

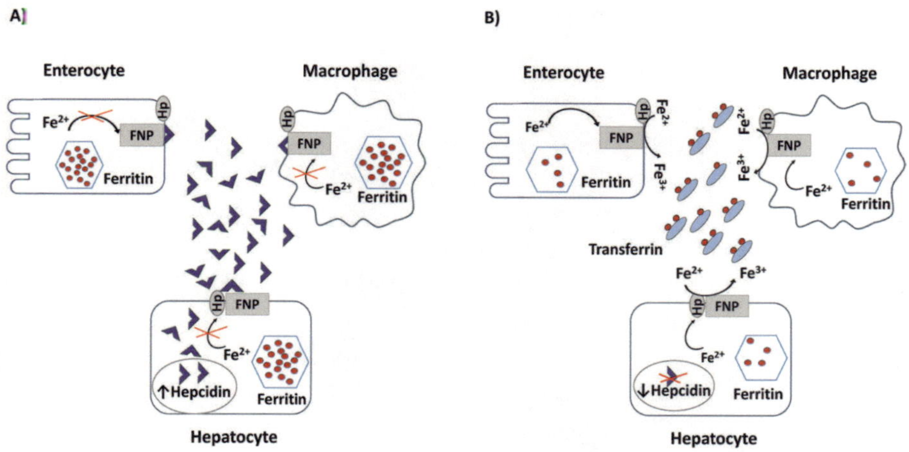

Figure 1. Role of hepcidin in systemic iron homeostasis. (A) High iron level conditions. Hepatic hepcidin expression and circulating hepcidin levels are increased; in hepatocytes, enterocytes, and macrophages, hepcidin is bound to the complex ferroportin-hephaestin and ferroportin is internalized and degraded; consequently, iron efflux is inhibited. (B) Low iron level conditions. Hepatic hepcidin synthesis is inhibited and serum hepcidin levels are negligible; consequently, iron crosses the membrane and is delivered into the circulation and transported to tissues by transferrin that is highly saturated (FNP: ferroportin; HP: hephaestin). Modified from Blanco-Rojo R. [24].

On the other hand, hepcidin regulation is a very active field. Many stimuli affect hepcidin transcription; the main factors are iron level, as explained above; inflammation, as hepcidin behaves as an acute phase protein; hypoxia, through the hypoxia inducible factor; and erythropoiesis signals. The details of hepcidin regulation and intracellular iron regulatory proteins involved in transcription are far beyond this revision and have been reviewed by others [16, 19, 24–27].

1.2. Role of macrophages in iron recycling

Hemoglobin in erythrocytes constitutes the major iron pool of the body. Senescent or damaged erythrocytes are phagocytosed by macrophages in the spleen, bone marrow, and liver. This activity is very efficient, as daily 20–25 mg of iron is delivered from macrophages into circulation and recycled, and the amount of iron that has to be absorbed for body functions is only 1–2 mg per day. Moreover, macrophages can work as a reservoir and participate in iron homeostasis [11].

Figure 2 shows the erythrophagocytic activity of macrophages. Once the macrophage detects an alteration or damage in the erythrocyte, the phagocytosis process is triggered. First, the erythrocyte is incorporated into the phagosome and heme is released. Then, heme is catabolized by hemoxigenase-1, and carbon monoxide, biliverdin, and Fe^{2+} are released. Fe^{2+} is transported across the phagosome membrane by DMT1 and natural resistance-associated

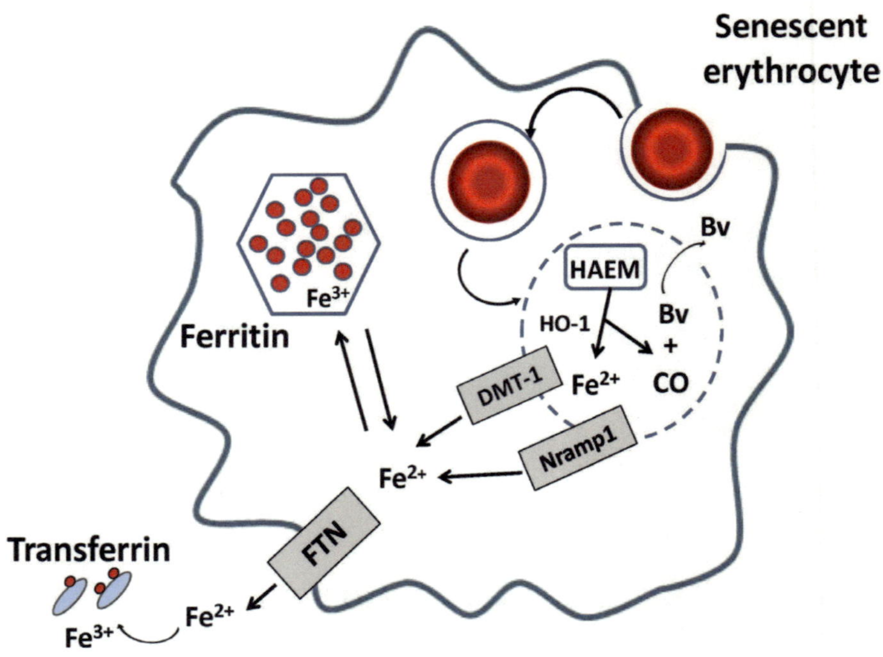

Figure 2. Erythrophagocytic activity of macrophages. CO: carbon monoxide; HO-1: hemoxygenase-1; Bv: biliverdin; DMT-1: dimetal transporter-1; Nramp1: natural resistance-associated macrophage protein; FTN: ferroportin. Modified from Blanco-Rojo R. [24].

macrophage protein (Nramp1). It seems that the presence of both transporters makes recycling more efficient. If iron is not needed for erythropoiesis, it is stored as ferritin in the form of Fe^{3+}. Finally, iron is released into the circulation via ferroportin and hephaestin (HP), and the iron is donated to transferrin to be reutilized [28].

2. Role of iron in oxidative status

The redox potential of iron, that is the switch between Fe^{2+} and Fe^{3+}, is essential for many biochemical reactions but is also a potential threat. Iron toxicity is based on the Fenton and Haber-Weiss reaction, which generates •OH (hydroxyl radicals) from H_2O_2 (hydrogen peroxide) and superoxide ($\bullet O_2^-$) in the presence of catalytic amounts of iron. The first step of the catalytic cycle involves reduction of ferric ion to ferrous:

$$Fe^{3+} + \bullet O_2^{\ -} \rightarrow Fe^{2+} + O_2 \tag{1}$$

The second step is:

$$Fe^{2+} + H_2O_2 \rightarrow Fe^{3+} + OH^- + \bullet OH \tag{2}$$

Net reaction:

$$\bullet O_2^{\ -} + H_2O_2 \rightarrow \bullet OH + OH^- + O_2 \,(\text{where Fe acts as a catalytic metal}) \tag{3}$$

The catalytic action of iron also leads to the formation of organic reactive oxygen species (ROS), such as peroxyl radicals (ROO•), alkoxyl radicals (RO•), thiyl radicals (RS•), sulfonyl radicals (ROS•), thiyl peroxyl radicals (RSOO•), and disulfides (RSSR). Similarly, heme iron catalyzes the formation of ROS, via the formation of oxoferryl intermediates. In addition, ferrous iron can also contribute as a reactant to free radical generation [29].

It is worth mentioning that ROS are normally produced by the mitochondria aerobic metabolism through the incomplete reduction of molecular oxygen. ROS can also be generated by the membrane-bound NADPH oxidase complex that is an important tool for the antimicrobial defense and is mainly expressed not only in phagocytic macrophages but also in neutrophils and other cell types.

ROS are highly reactive species and promote the oxidation of proteins, nucleic acids, and membrane lipids. Any increase in the ROS levels beyond the antioxidant capacity of the organism causes oxidative stress [29]. In this regard, in primary and secondary iron overload conditions, such as in hereditary hemochromatosis and thalassemia, respectively, oxidative stress is observed as the iron-binding capacity of transferrin gets saturated and high levels of non-transferrin-bound iron reach the cell, are internalized, and induce tissue damage [30, 31].

Excess iron is involved in the pathophysiology of chronic inflammation, Alzheimer disease, diabetes, atherosclerosis, and, generally, cardiovascular diseases (CVD).

3. Iron excess and cardiovascular risk

3.1. The iron hypothesis

Early in the 1980s, Sullivan published in *The Lancet* the hypothesis that higher-stored iron in men and postmenopausal women compared to premenopausal women increase the risk of heart diseases and that iron deficiency is a protective factor [32]. This was supported by epidemiological studies; positive associations between serum ferritin (marker of iron stores), and the cholesterol transported by low-density lipoproteins (LDL-cholesterol) that were reported in men [33]. But other data do not support this hypothesis [34, 35] and the debate still continues. Our research group and others have reported that iron-deficient and anemic women present low lipid levels that increase during pharmacological treatment with iron salts, although final values are in normal range [36, 37]. Other studies coincide in the gender and age differences in iron metabolism and lipoprotein metabolism and the lower cardiovascular risk in women compared to men [38]. However, there may be several interacting factors. In this regard, estrogens are related to higher levels of cholesterol transported by high-density lipoproteins (HDL-cholesterol) and aldosterone that may partly explain lower atherosclerosis and hypertension risk [39]. However, age has been suggested to exert higher influence than hormones as estrogens explain about 25% of the phenotype differences related to cardiovascular risk, and thus menopausal women have higher cardiovascular risk than fertile women mainly due to age [40]. Studies in older men and women do not support the Sullivan's hypothesis and are rather opposite, with a subgroup of individuals who have low iron stores and higher cardiovascular risk [41]. Likewise, our findings in an elderly population consuming a variant of the Mediterranean diet show that prevalence of anemia is higher than that of high ferritin [42].

Therefore, it is likely that iron is only one of the players in the pathophysiological process of cardiovascular diseases.

3.2. Iron excess and atherosclerosis

Atherosclerosis is a chronic inflammatory disease affecting the arterial intima [43, 44]. Endothelial dysfunction induces recruitment of LDL particles and blood monocytes that differentiate into macrophages, phagocyte lipid material, and are transformed into foam cells [45]. The possibility that iron plays an interacting role emerges from its capacity to enhance the formation of ROS and LDL oxidation and its presence in macrophages, where a reservoir of intracellular iron may remain if body iron is high. In this regard, high iron levels hypothetically increase atherosclerosis risk.

However, there are many doubts on this hypothesis. Results from the ARIC study, carried out in the 1990s, did not find an association between ferritin values and LDL oxidation [43] or ferritin and asymptomatic carotid atherosclerosis [44]. Likewise, a recent systematic analysis by Hosseini [46] concludes that iron intake/status is not associated with carotid intima media thickness. In this issue, it could be speculated that the effect of iron is related to the "labile pool" or unbound iron more than to the total amount of iron in the body.

Results from the MONICA study in France [47] show that carotid atherosclerosis was positively associated with serum ferritin in individuals free from subclinical inflammation. In another study [48], atherosclerotic plaque specimens, which were removed from carotids of patients as a stroke reduction strategy, were analyzed. The study compared symptomatic and asymptomatic plaques considering that stroke symptoms occur when carotid bifurcation plaque ruptures and clots move into the cerebral circulation. It has been assumed that iron accumulates in atherosclerosis plaques following plaque rupture and hemorrhage since phagocytosed erythrocytes have been identified in plaque macrophages. It was found that in the symptomatic plaque (causing stenosis and cerebrovascular symptoms), iron is associated with the patient's LDL-cholesterol level. Furthermore, iron is abundant in such unstable plaques within thrombus, in the presence of macrophages, and away from calcium and zinc, elements that co-localize in areas of plaque mineralization. Finally, iron in asymptomatic plaque (causing stenosis but not neurological symptoms) was present as ferritin and was observed in association with CD68-positive macrophages.

Therefore, iron may be involved both in the initial step of atherosclerosis by activating LDL oxidation and in the final step linked to the vessel lesion within the plaque. Interestingly, increasing the iron levels in circulating macrophages do not increase atherosclerosis [49]. In a mouse model of atherosclerosis (ApoE-/-), mice were fed with a high-fat diet and their tissue iron was increased by parenteral iron administration and a genetic mutation in ferroportin [49]. Iron loading produced an iron level increase in macrophages, liver, and spleen and resulted in the activation of the macrophage antioxidant defenses and in the storage of iron in the form of ferritin. Clearly, this regulation reduced NTBI and toxicity.

With the hypothesis that blood donation reduces cardiovascular risk by lowering body iron status, a study was done in 819 healthy blood donors in the Netherlands [50]. Data included blood donation frequency, body iron status parameters, and a measure of the carotid intima-media thickness (CIMT). Body iron status was not related to CIMT, but CIMT was slightly and not significantly reduced in frequent donors. Therefore, blood donation might give some protection against atherosclerosis in individuals predisposed to accumulate iron in excess, but the mechanism may be independent of total body iron.

The possibility that heme instead of iron is the inductor of LDL oxidation has also been investigated [51, 52]. Heme oxygenase-1, the heme-catabolizing enzyme, is therefore crucial for heme detoxification (see HO-1 in **Figure 2**). HO-1 induction results in an increase in free iron and ferritin upregulation, which means iron storage and protection of the cell [51]. Interestingly, a child with HO-1 deficiency showed elevated plasma heme levels, extensive LDL oxidation, severe endothelial damage, and accelerated atherosclerosis, and thus the possibility of a HO-1 therapy that mitigates some of the symptoms is a matter of research [52, 53].

3.3. Lessons from hemochromatosis and other iron overload disturbances

Type 1 hereditary hemochromatosis (HH) is a genetic disease defined as homozygous for the C282Y mutation of the *HFE* gene. This gene is located in chromosome 6 and encodes the major histocompatibility complex class I-like protein HFE. The prevalence of HH is approximately 0.1% in the population of Caucasian origin. However, low morbidity has been found in HH and most of the C282Y +/+ have no iron overload phenotype or are asymptomatic until adulthood. Cash et al. [30] compared vascular function, biochemical endothelial markers, and antioxidant status between HH patients (C282Y homozygous and high serum-ferritin levels) and controls. Noninvasive pulse wave analysis and pulse wave velocity were applied to carotid and radial arteries to estimate endothelial dysfunction. They reported that male HH patients had higher pulse wave velocity; however, this effect disappeared after adjusting for hypertension. In both sexes, HH was associated with diminished antioxidant levels but neither increase in lipid peroxidation nor alteration in the systemic inflammation marker (i.e., C-reactive protein) could be demonstrated [30]. Thus, controversy remains on the idea that cardiovascular risk is high in hemochromatosis patients [54].

Iron overload is usually a complication of thalassemia, particularly in patients who require red blood cell transfusions. Among the three types of thalassemia, thalassemia intermedia is characterized by ineffective erythropoiesis, anemia, medullary expansion, and extramedullary hematopoiesis. In contrast to HH, thalassemic patients show a proatherogenic biochemical phenotype which may contribute to enhance cardiovascular risks [31].

There are other iron overload pathological situations, where bone medulla is inefficient and iron overload results from repeated transfusions. In such syndromes, the amount of body iron can reach very high values and myocardial damage is the most frequent collateral effect of the treatment. In these cases, iron chelation therapy may result in higher quality of life and reduction of cardiac events [55].

4. Iron deficiency anemia and cardiovascular risk

Oxidative stress results from disequilibrium between oxidants and antioxidants. While iron excess may be involved in the generation of ROS, as commented above, anemia due to iron deficiency anemia (IDA) may affect the functioning of many enzymatic systems (cytochromes, catalases, hydroxylases, etc.) related to immunity, antioxidant status, and DNA integrity, among others [56].

In this regard, Aslan et al. [57] compared total plasma antioxidant capacity and lymphocyte DNA damage between two groups of IDA and control adults and concluded that both oxidative stress and DNA damage increased in IDA. In another study, four groups were compared: patients recently diagnosed with IDA who were not receiving any treatment at the beginning of the study; patients with IDA at the sixth week of an iron-replacement program (considered the time of hemoglobin normalization); patients with IDA at the end of the iron-replacement treatment (time of saturation of body iron stores); and age- and sex-matched healthy controls. Results show that untreated IDA patients present high lipid peroxidation, assessed by plasma malondialdehyde, and low activities of the antioxidant enzymes glutathione peroxidase, superoxide dismutase, and catalase and that the values did not differ between the sixth week and the end of the treatment, suggesting that recovery from IDA reduces oxidative stress [58]. Unfortunately, in these studies, the changes within a patient were not analyzed. In animal models of IDA, where all experimental conditions are controlled, high oxidative stress and DNA damage were not demonstrated [59, 60].

Another aspect that has been studied is the possible changes in lipid levels in IDA. Old animal studies reported dyslipidemia with altered triglycerides and total cholesterol in serum. However, in most animal experiments, there were important confounders. For instance, iron deficiency induces low appetite and a reduction in food intake that often was not adequately controlled. In this regard, there are inconsistent results, but clearly the direction of change was toward reduction in circulating lipids and profound modifications in lipoprotein metabolism [61].

In humans, our research group found low values of total cholesterol, HDL-cholesterol, glucose, and uric acid in IDA women at fertile age, which significantly increased during anemia recovery [36]. These results coincide with that of others who also reported low serum triglycerides [62] and LDL-cholesterol [63]. It is noteworthy that despite significant increases after treatment, the observed lipid values were very low in the severe anemic patients from these studies and still did not reach levels of non-anemic controls after recovery (reported mean values were approximately 150–170 mg/dL for total cholesterol and 60–70 mg/dL for triglycerides).

The above results can be explained by inhibition of lipid biosynthesis due to iron deficiency. Kamei et al. [64] performed a transcriptome analysis to determine the effects of iron deficiency on hepatic gene expression. Rats on an iron-deficient diet were compared with rats pair-fed a control diet with a normal iron level. In agreement with human studies, these authors observed that iron deficiency decreases cholesterol and triglycerides in serum and liver. In addition, they found that serum glucose and insulin increased. Expressions of genes encoding gluconeogenic enzymes were upregulated, lactate was increased, and the urea cycle was activated. These results are explained by the insufficiency of iron for its enzymatic functions and the situation of hypoxia due to anemia. Nevertheless, the results of high glucose and insulin do not agree with human observations.

Iron deficiency may affect cardiovascular health by indirect mechanisms. In this regard, iron participates in the hydroxylation of vitamin D to the active metabolites, 25 hydroxyvitamin D and 1,25-hydroxyvitamin D, and vitamin D acts as an antioxidant and may have protective cardiovascular effects, decreasing LDL-cholesterol, and blood pressure [37]. Moreover, iron supplementation alone increases vitamin B12 and folic acid levels [36]. This is attributed to a general increase in intestinal mucosa that favors nutrient absorption.

5. Dysmetabolic iron, type 2 diabetes, and cardiometabolic alterations

5.1. Iron excess and type 2 diabetes mellitus (T2DM)

T2DM is the most common and an ever-increasing form of diabetes [65]. It is characterized by disorders in insulin secretion or action either of which maybe the predominant feature. The association between iron overload and T2DM came from the observation that the frequency of diabetes is increased in classic hereditary hemochromatosis [65]. A link between red meat consumption, one of the highest iron bioavailability source, and T2DM has been reported [66]. Moreover, some reports show a relationship between high ferritin and the risk of gestational diabetes [67].

The positive association between iron excess and T2DM is feasible although the underlying mechanisms still remain to be fully determined. First, iron is a powerful pro-oxidant and catalyst molecule, which promotes the formation of hydroxyl radicals and could attack pancreatic β cells by increasing oxidative stress thus resulting in impaired insulin synthesis and secretion [68]. Second, iron excess can diminish insulin utilization in muscle tissue leading to a shift from glucose to free acid oxidation, which may result in enhanced insulin resistance [69]. Third, increasing free fatty acid, main substrate for hepatic gluconeogenesis, would provoke higher glucose production [69]. Thus, the possible mechanisms are insulin deficiency, insulin resistance, and hepatic dysfunction [70].

Several studies report an association between the heme iron intake and risk of T2DM. The prospective cohort within the Nurses' Health Study found that higher intake of heme iron was associated with higher intake of fat (total and saturated), red meat, and protein and with lower intake of carbohydrates. However, the association was not entirely explained by the red meat intake. Total dietary iron, non-heme iron, or supplemental iron were not related to diabetes risk [71].

Other studies reveal that vegetarians have higher insulin sensitivity than omnivores, and this was mainly attributed to their lower body iron [72]. In this regard, blood donation, by reducing iron stores, may increase insulin sensitivity [72, 73]. However, there is controversy in this issue [74–76].

We have studied some cardiovascular risk markers in a population of 595 T2DM from the DIabetes and CArdiovascular RIsk VAllecas (DICARIVA) study according to ferritin levels (**Table 1**).

Diabetic dyslipidemia is a cluster of altered plasma lipids and lipoproteins [77] though LDL-cholesterol levels are normal or reduced. It is characterized by high triglycerides and low HDL-cholesterol levels and by increased number of small and dense LDL particles [77]. Altogether, these features are known as the lipidic triad. In addition, other alterations are often observed:

- Increased concentration of very low density lipoproteins (VLDL) due to an increased production or a lower clearance of triglycerides and apolipoprotein (apo) B.
- Increased production of apo B-LDL as well as an increment in glycosylation and oxidation of LDL particles.

	n	Mean	Standard deviation	P25	Median	P75
Males	265	150.5	149.3	50.5	107	200.5
Females	330	67.6	83	21.8	41.5	78

The distribution of ferritin in male and femaleT2DM was significantly different ($p < 0.0001$).

Table 1. Male and female ferritin levels (ng/mL) in type 2 diabetes population belonging to the DIabetes and CArdiovascular RIsk VAllecas (DICARIVA) study P25 and P75, 25th and 75th percentiles.

- Higher clearance of apo A1 with decrease in the high-size HDLs and decrease of the cholesterol reverse transport.
- Lower clearance of chylomicrons and remnant particles (i.e., intermedium density lipoproteins or IDL).

The diabetic dyslipidemia is associated with insulin resistance, visceral obesity, and liver fat content. Furthermore, insulin resistance is related to an excessive flux of substrates (free fatty acids and glucose) to participate in the formation of VLDL in the liver and with a positive control of mechanisms that produces an excess of large VLDL. These lipoprotein metabolism anomalies are not disconnected facts but are closely related to each other [78]. It is known that lipid metabolism in T2DM is modulated by several factors, such as the degree of glucose control and insulin resistance. The hypertriglyceridemia is very prevalent in T2DM and is also frequent in prediabetes, preceding the presence of chronic hyperglycemia [79]. When there is insulin resistance, mesenteric or "central" adipocytes are full and are unable to retain more fatty acids, consequently fatty acids reach the liver in very high quantities.

Since LDL-size assessment requires special methodology, other approaches have been proposed. The triglycerides/HDL-cholesterol molar ratio has been widely used as a surrogate marker of LDL-size in clinical practice [80]. Earlier a value < 1.33 for this ratio was considered adequate and indicative of large LDL particles. In contrast, individuals with high triglyceride/LDL-cholesterol molar ratio present a high amount of small, dense, oxidizable, and, thus, highly atherogenic LDL particles [81].

It has been confirmed that triglyceridemia is the determinant of LDL size [82]. In fact, it has been proposed that highly enriched in triglyceride VLDL subtype (VLDL1) are the predecessors of dense and small LDL particles [83].

According to the data in **Table 2**, T2DM women presented higher triglyceridemia and higher HDL-cholesterol levels but lower triglyceride/HDL-cholesterol levels than men.

This study also shows that triglyceride levels increase in parallel to the level of ferritin in men and women. Triglycerides were 36 and 23% higher in men and women, respectively, belonging to the 4th ferritin quartile *versus* their 1st counterparts. LDL particles appear 38% smaller in men and 24% smaller in women at the highest quartile *versus* the lowest, according to the triglyceride/HDL-cholesterol molar ratio. Taking into account these data and the significant correlation between ferritin and this molar ratio ($p < 0.001$), it can be speculated that body iron contributes to this theoretically higher oxidability and atherogenicity of the LDL.

When the T2DM sample belonging to the 1st or 4th quartile for ferritin was stratified according to the presence of normo or hypertriglyceridemia, low or high levels of HDL-cholesterol, and small or large LDL particles, it was observed that the prevalence of altered triglycerides was higher (odd ratio 1.78; $p=0.011$) in T2DM patients belonging to the highest quartile for ferritin. Similarly, the odd ratios for high levels of HDL-cholesterol or the presence of small LDLs was 0.54 ($p = 0.010$) and 1.93 ($p = 0.004$), respectively in the T2DM patients of the 4th quartile *versus* the 1st quartile of ferritin.

To insist even more in this idea, the prevalence of T2DM presenting the lipid triad was compared to that of patients who did not present any of the three components of the triad. The

		Ferritin quartiles	N	Mean	SD	95% CI Lower limit	95% CI Upper limit	ANOVA *p*	P25 *vs* P75
Men	Triglycerides	<P25	66	128.6	63.1	113.0	144.1	0.038	0.006
	mg/dL	P25-<P75	133	157.8	114.3	138.2	177.4		
		≥P75	66	174.8	118.5	145.7	203.9		
	HDL-cholesterol	<P25	66	48.4	12.5	45.3	51.5	0.99	0.96
	mg/dL	P25-<P75	133	48.6	12.7	46.4	50.7		
		≥P75	66	48.2	12.5	45.4	51.5		
	TG/HDLc*	<P25	66	1.29	0.82	1.08	1.49	0.013	0.020
	mol/mol	P25-<P75	133	1.63	1.66	1.35	1.92		
		≥P75	66	1.78	1.47	1.42	2.14		
Women	Triglycerides	<P25	82	152.8	95.4	131.9	173.8	0.027	0.17
	mg/dL	P25-<P75	163	138.1	101.6	122.4	153.8		
		≥P75	84	187.9	213.1	141.7	234.2		
	HDL-cholesterol	<P25	82	59.2	14.9	55.9	62.4	0.025	0.007
	mg/dL	P25-<P75	163	56.5	14.1	54.3	58.7		
		≥P75	84	53.2	13.3	50.3	56.1		
	TG/HDLc*	<P25	82	1.33	1.20	1.07	1.59	0.038	0.11
	mol/mol	P25-<P75	163	1.21	1.27	1.01	1.41		
		≥P75	84	1.65	1.40	1.35	1.96		

P, percentile; ANOVA *p*, P value for <P25, P25-<75 and ≥P75.

*TG/HDLc, Triglycerides/HDL-cholesterol molar ratio.

Table 2. Triglyceride, HDL-cholesterol, and the Triglyceride/HDL-cholesterol molar ratio in men and women from the DIabetes and CArdiovascular RIsk VAllecas (DICARIVA) study stratified according to ferritin quartiles.

concurrence of high ferritin and all the three components of the triad was higher than the concurrence of low ferritin and the three components of the triad. On the contrary, the absence of any of the three components of the triad was less prevalent in T2DM patients with high ferritin values than in their low ferritin counterparts. The odd ratio for the lipid triad/ferritin association was 2.23 ($p = 0.010$), suggesting the hypothesis that altered CVD risk factors is more prevalent in T2DM patients presenting high iron body stores.

6. Conclusions, remarks, and future research

From all the above, there clearly exists a connection between iron regulation, lipoprotein metabolism, and insulin resistance.

Experimental evidence in animals and humans indicates that dietary fat may be important in iron metabolism. Despite increasing evidence that dietary fat can influence iron absorption and retention, there is a paucity of information about the mechanism implicated [84, 85]. These may be related directly to changes occurring within the intestinal lumen in the enterocytes at luminal or apical membranes. Many aspects of iron absorption and its regulation are still unknown, such as the mechanisms of ferric iron transport, the role of mucines, and so on [8, 9, 11].

Droke et al. [86] demonstrate that palmitate increased iron transport to a greater extent than stearate, and this is followed by far by oleate, which could be due to fatty acid metabolism within the cells and the elongation of palmitic to stearic acid. However, the results suggest that fatty acids affected iron uptake to a greater extent than iron transport. One of the most striking effects of dietary fat on mineral metabolism is the finding of the enhancement of iron uptake and utilization by saturated fat. The effects are prominent when dietary iron is limiting and thus indicate a novel role in promoting an adequate iron status in human [86].

A genome-wide association study (GWA study or GWAS) and epigenome-wide association study (EWAS) together with metabolomic studies would help much to understand the mechanisms involved in the conjoint iron-lipid metabolism that, in turn, affects CVD risks. This information will be useful in the dietary personalization to optimize human health and function.

Meanwhile, as saturated fatty acids (mainly palmitic) increase the iron store [86], total cholesterol, and LDL cholesterol, and induce negative effects on insulin resistance compared to unsaturated fat [87], the authors of the present review claim insisting in the need that T2DM patients show a high adherence to present dietary recommendations for diabetes (American Diabetes Association [88]), which textually include that fat quality (eating monounsaturated and polyunsaturated fats and avoiding *trans* fats and saturated fats) appears to be more important than quantity.

In conclusion, iron is a key metal involved in cardiovascular health. Mild iron deficiency may reduce cardiovascular risk; contrarily, severe anemia induces alterations in the antioxidant iron-dependent enzymes and can be a threat. Iron overload appears to be more important than deficiency in triggering insulin resistance. In this regard, dysmetabolic iron overload syndrome has been related to liver fat accumulation and visceral adiposity [89]. Whether hepcidin resistance is linked to insulin resistance should be a matter of further research.

Our data in an ample sample of adults diagnosed with T2DM suggest that body iron stores, evaluated as serum ferritin, are clearly related with some key markers of the so-called lipidic triad of the T2DM (high triglyceride and low HDL-cholesterol levels together with the presence of small and dense LDL particles) which also is in the frame of the dysmetabolic iron overload syndrome.

Acknowledgements

This study was partially supported by the Spanish project AGL2014-53207-C2-2-R. We also acknowledge type 2 diabetes mellitus patients from de DICARIVA study for their voluntary participation and the Infanta Leonor Hospital of Madrid (Spain).

Abbreviations

CVD	cardiovascular diseases
DMT1	divalent metal transporter
FPN	ferroportin
IDA	iron deficiency anemia
HDL-cholesterol	cholesterol transported by high density lipoproteins
NTBI	non-transferrin-bound iron
ROS	reactive oxygen species
T2DM	type 2 diabetes mellitus
TfR1	transferrin receptor

Author details

María Pilar Vaquero[1], Ángel García-Quismondo[2], Francisco J. del Cañizo[3*] and Francisco J. Sánchez-Muniz[2]

*Address all correspondence to: frasan@ucm.es

1 Department of Metabolism and Nutrition, Institute of Food Science, Technology and Nutrition, Spanish National Research Council (ICTAN-CSIC), Madrid, Spain

2 Department of Nutrition, Universidad Complutense de Madrid, Madrid, Spain

3 Servicio de Endocrinología, Hospital Infanta Leonor, Madrid, Spain

References

[1] Toxqui L, De Piero A, Courtois V, Bastida S, Sanchez-Muniz FJ, Vaquero MP. Iron deficiency and overload. Implications in oxidative stress and cardiovascular health. Nutricion Hospitalaria. 2010;**25**(3):350-365

[2] Hare DJ, Double KL. Iron and dopamine: A toxic couple. Brain. 2016;**139**(Pt 4):1026-1035

[3] Blanco-Rojo R, Perez-Granados AM, Toxqui L, Gonzalez-Vizcayno C, Delgado MA, Vaquero MP. Efficacy of a microencapsulated iron pyrophosphate-fortified fruit juice: A randomized, double-blind, placebo-controlled study in Spanish iron-deficient women. The British Journal of Nutrition 2011;**105**(11):1652-1659

[4] Navas-Carretero S, Perez-Granados AM, Sarria B, Carbajal A, Pedrosa MM, Roe MA, et al. Oily fish increases iron bioavailability of a phytate rich meal in young iron deficient women. Journal of the American College of Nutrition. 2008;**27**(1):96-101

[5] Navas-Carretero S, Perez-Granados AM, Sarria B, Vaquero MP. Iron absorption from meat pate fortified with ferric pyrophosphate in iron-deficient women. Nutrition. 2009;**25**(1):20-24

[6] Navas-Carretero S, Perez-Granados AM, Schoppen S, Sarria B, Carbajal A, Vaquero MP. Iron status biomarkers in iron deficient women consuming oily fish versus red meat diet. Journal of Physiology and Biochemistry. 2009;**65**(2):165-174

[7] Toxqui L, Perez-Granados AM, Blanco-Rojo R, Wright I, Gonzalez-Vizcayno C, Vaquero MP. Effects of an iron or iron and vitamin D-fortified flavored skim milk on iron metabolism: A randomized controlled double-blind trial in iron-deficient women. Journal of the American College of Nutrition. 2013;**32**(5):312-320

[8] Chamorro S, Gutierrez L, Vaquero MP, Verdoy D, Salas G, Luengo Y, et al. Safety assessment of chronic oral exposure to iron oxide nanoparticles. Nanotechnology. 2015;**26**(20):205101

[9] Sharp PA. Intestinal iron absorption: Regulation by dietary & systemic factors. International Journal for Vitamin and Nutrition Research. 2010;**80**(4-5):231-242

[10] Alwan NA, Hamamy H. Maternal iron status in pregnancy and long-term health outcomes in the offspring. Journal of Pediatric Genetics. 2015;**4**(2):111-123

[11] Garrick MD, Garrick LM. Cellular iron transport. Biochimica et Biophysica Acta (BBA)—General Subjects. 2009;**1790**(5):309-325

[12] Toxqui L, Perez-Granados AM, Blanco-Rojo R, Wright I, Vaquero MP. A simple and feasible questionnaire to estimate menstrual blood loss: Relationship with hematological and gynecological parameters in young women. BMC Womens Health. 2014;**14**:71

[13] Lane DJR, Merlot AM, Huang MLH, Bae DH, Jansson PJ, Sahni S, et al. Cellular iron uptake, trafficking and metabolism: Key molecules and mechanisms and their roles in disease. Biochimica et Biophysica Acta (BBA)—Molecular Cell Research. 2015;**1853**(5):1130-1144

[14] Krause A, Neitz S, Mägert H-J, Schulz A, Forssmann W-G, Schulz-Knappe P, et al. LEAP-1, a novel highly disulfide-bonded human peptide, exhibits antimicrobial activity. FEBS Letters. 2000;**480**(2-3):147-150

[15] Park CH, Valore EV, Waring AJ, Ganz T. Hepcidin, a urinary antimicrobial peptide synthesized in the liver. The Journal of Biological Chemistry. 2001;**276**(11):7806

[16] Schmidt PJ. Regulation of iron metabolism by hepcidin under conditions of inflammation. The Journal of Biological Chemistry. 2015;**290**(31):18975-18983

[17] Sarriá B, López-Parra AM, Navas-Carretero S, Pérez-Granados AM, Baeza C, Arroyo-Pardo E, et al. Hepcidin, transferrin (exon 7), and hemochromatosis genotyping suggests that haplotype block analysis is the best strategy for predicting iron deficiency phenotype in women. Nutrition Research. 2007;**27**(11):672-678

[18] Roetto A, Papanikolaou G, Politou M, Alberti F, Girelli D, Christakis J, et al. Mutant antimicrobial peptide hepcidin is associated with severe juvenile hemochromatosis. Nature Genetics. 2003;**33**(1):21-22

[19] Blanco-Rojo R, Baeza-Richer C, Lopez-Parra AM, Perez-Granados AM, Brichs A, Bertoncini S, et al. Four variants in transferrin and HFE genes as potential markers of iron deficiency anemia risk: An association study in menstruating women. Nutrition and Metabolism(London). 2011;**8**:69

[20] Blanco-Rojo R, Bayele HK, Srai SK, Vaquero MP. Intronic SNP rs3811647 of the human transferrin gene modulates its expression in hepatoma cells. Nutrición Hospitalaria. 2012;**27**(6):2142-2145

[21] Baeza-Richer C, Arroyo-Pardo E, Blanco-Rojo R, Toxqui L, Remacha A, Vaquero MP, et al. Genetic contribution to iron status: SNPs related to iron deficiency anemia and fine mapping of CACNA2D3 calcium channel subunit. Blood Cells, Molecules, and Diseases. 2015;**55**(4):273-280

[22] Baeza-Richer C, Blanco-Rojo R, Lopez-Parra AM, Brichs A, Bertoncini S, Perez-Granados AM, et al. Identification of a novel quantitative trait nucleotype related to iron status in a calcium channel gene. Disease Markers. 2013;**34**(2):121-129

[23] Sarria B, Navas-Carretero S, Lopez-Parra AM, Perez-Granados AM, Arroyo-Pardo E, Roe MA, et al. The G277S transferrin mutation does not affect iron absorption in iron deficient women. European Journal of Nutrition. 2007;**46**(1):57-60

[24] Blanco-Rojo R. Dietary, genetic and physiological risk factors for iron deficiency anemia, and efficacy of a functional food in iron deficient women [thesis]. Madrid: Complutense University; 2012

[25] Ganz T. Hepcidin and iron regulation, 10 years later. Blood. 2011;**117**(17):4425-4433

[26] Liu J, Sun B, Yin H, Liu S. Hepcidin: A promising therapeutic target for iron disorders: A systematic review. Medicine. 2016;**95**(14):e3150

[27] Arezes J, Nemeth E. Hepcidin and iron disorders: New biology and clinical approaches. International Journal of Laboratory Hematology. 2015;**37**(Suppl 1):92-98

[28] Soe-Lin S, Apte SS, Mikhael MR, Kayembe LK, Nie G, Ponka P. Both Nramp1 and DMT1 are necessary for efficient macrophage iron recycling. Experimental Hematology. 2010;**38**(8):609-617

[29] Papanikolaou G, Pantopoulos K. Iron metabolism and toxicity. Toxicology and Applied Pharmacology. 2005;**202**(2):199-211

[30] Cash WJ, O'Neill S, O'Donnell ME, McCance DR, Young IS, McEneny J, et al. Disordered vascular compliance in haemochromatosis. Irish Journal of Medical Science. 2014;**183**(2):303-309

[31] Lai ME, Vacquer S, Carta MP, Spiga A, Cocco P, Angius F, et al. Thalassemia intermedia is associated with a proatherogenic biochemical phenotype. Blood Cells, Molecules & Diseases. 2011;**46**(4):294-299

[32] Sullivan J. Iron and the sex difference in heart disease risk. The Lancet. 1981;**317**(8233): 1293-1294

[33] Salonen JT, Nyyssönen K, Korpela H, Tuomilehto J, Seppänen R, Salonen R. High stored iron levels are associated with excess risk of myocardial infarction in eastern Finnish men. Circulation. 1992;**86**(3):803

[34] Sempos CT, Looker AC. Iron status and the risk of coronary heart disease: An example of the use of nutritional epidemiology in chronic disease research. Journal of Nutritional Biochemistry. 2001;**12**(3):170-182

[35] Corti MC, Gaziano M, Hennekens CH. Iron status and risk of cardiovascular disease. Annals of Epidemiology. 1997;**7**:7

[36] Remacha AF, Wright I, Fernandez-Jimenez MC, Toxqui L, Blanco-Rojo R, Moreno G, et al. Vitamin B12 and folate levels increase during treatment of iron deficiency anaemia in young adult woman. International Journal of Laboratory Hematology. 2015;**37**(5):641-648

[37] Toxqui L, Blanco-Rojo R, Wright I, Perez-Granados AM, Vaquero MP. Changes in blood pressure and lipid levels in young women consuming a vitamin D-fortified skimmed milk: A randomised controlled trial. Nutrients. 2013;**5**(12):4966-4977

[38] Klip IT, Voors AA, Swinkels DW, Bakker SJ, Kootstra-Ros JE, Lam CS, et al. Serum ferritin and risk for new-onset heart failure and cardiovascular events in the community. European Journal of Heart Failure. 2016;**19**:348-356

[39] Toxqui L, Vaquero MP. Aldosterone changes after consumption of a sodium-bicarbonated mineral water in humans. A four-way randomized controlled trial. Journal of Physiology and Biochemistry. 2016;**72**(4):635-641

[40] Casiglia E, Tikhonoff V, Caffi S, Bascelli A, Schiavon L, Guidotti F, et al. Menopause does not affect blood pressure and risk profile, and menopausal women do not become similar to men. Journal of Hypertension. 2008;**26**(10):1983-1992

[41] Corti M-C, Guralnik JM, Salive ME, Ferrucci L, Pahor M, Wallace RB, et al. Serum iron level, coronary artery disease, and all-cause mortality in older men and women. American Journal of Cardiology. 1997;**79**(2):120-127

[42] Vaquero MP, Sanchez-Muniz FJ, Carbajal A, Garcia-Linares MC, Garcia-Fernandez MC, Garcia-Arias MT. Mineral and vitamin status in elderly persons from Northwest Spain consuming an Atlantic variant of the Mediterranean diet. Annals of Nutrition & Metabolism. 2004;**48**(3):125-133

[43] Iribarren C, Sempos CT, Eckfeldt JH, Folsom AR. Lack of association between ferritin level and measures of LDL oxidation: The ARIC study. Atherosclerosis Risk in Communities. Atherosclerosis. 1998;**139**(1):189-195

[44] Moore M, Folsom AR, Barnes RW, Eckfeldt JH. No association between serum ferritin and asymptomatic carotid atherosclerosis. The Atherosclerosis Risk in Communities (ARIC) Study. American Journal of Epidemiology. 1995;**141**(8):719-723

[45] Moore KJ, Sheedy FJ, Fisher EA. Macrophages in atherosclerosis: A dynamic balance. Nature Reviews Immunology. 2013;**13**(10):709-721

[46] Hosseini B, Saedisomeolia A, Skilton MR. Association between micronutrients intake/status and carotid intima media thickness: A systematic review. Journal of the Academy of Nutrition and Dietetics. 2016;**117**:69-82

[47] Ahluwalia N, Genoux A, Ferrieres J, Perret B, Carayol M, Drouet L, et al. Iron status is associated with carotid atherosclerotic plaques in middle-aged adults. Journal of Nutrition. 2010;**140**(4):812-816

[48] Kopriva D, Kisheev A, Meena D, Pelle S, Karnitsky M, Lavoie A, et al. The nature of iron deposits differs between symptomatic and asymptomatic carotid atherosclerotic plaques. PLoS One. 2015;**10**(11):e0143138

[49] Kautz L, Gabayan V, Wang X, Wu J, Onwuzurike J, Jung G, et al. Testing the iron hypothesis in a mouse model of atherosclerosis. Cell Reports. 2013;**5**(5):1436-1442

[50] Engberink MF, Geleijnse JM, Durga J, Swinkels DW, de Kort WL, Schouten EG, et al. Blood donation, body iron status and carotid intima-media thickness. Atherosclerosis. 2008;**196**(2):856-862

[51] Hoekstra KA, Godin DV, Cheng KM. Protective role of heme oxygenase in the blood vessel wall during atherogenesis. Biochemistry and Cell Biology. 2004;**82**(3):351-359

[52] Jeney V, Balla J, Yachie A, Varga Z, Vercellotti GM, Eaton JW, et al. Pro-oxidant and cytotoxic effects of circulating heme. Blood. 2002;**100**(3):879-887

[53] Morita T. Heme oxygenase and atherosclerosis. Arteriosclerosis Thrombosis and Vascular Biology. 2005;**25**(9):1786-1795

[54] Mascitelli L, Goldstein MR. Hereditary hemochromatosis, iron, hepcidin, and coronary heart disease. Medical Hypotheses. 2014;**82**(3):402-403

[55] Remacha ÁF, Arrizabalaga B, Villegas A, Durán MS, Hermosín L, de Paz R, et al. Evolution of iron overload in patients with low-risk myelodysplastic syndrome: Iron chelation therapy and organ complications. Annals of Hematology. 2015;**94**(5):779-787

[56] Zhang C. Essential functions of iron-requiring proteins in DNA replication, repair and cell cycle control. Protein & Cell. 2014;**5**(10):750-760

[57] Aslan M, Horoz M, Kocyigit A, Ozgonul S, Celik H, Celik M, et al. Lymphocyte DNA damage and oxidative stress in patients with iron deficiency anemia. Mutation Research—Fundamental and Molecular Mechanisms of Mutagenesis. 2006;**601**(1-2):144-149

[58] Kurtoglu E, Ugur A, Baltaci AK, Undar L. Effect of iron supplementation on oxidative stress and antioxidant status in iron-deficiency anemia. Biological Trace Element Research. 2003;**96**(1):117-123

[59] Diaz-Castro J, Alferez MJ, Lopez-Aliaga I, Nestares T, Granados S, Barrionuevo M, et al. Influence of nutritional iron deficiency anemia on DNA stability and lipid peroxidation in rats. Nutrition. 2008;**24**(11-12):1167-1173

[60] Díaz-Castro J, Pérez-Sánchez LJ, Ramírez López-Frías M, López-Aliaga I, Nestares T, Alférez MJM, et al. Influence of cow or goat milk consumption on antioxidant defence and lipid peroxidation during chronic iron repletion. British Journal of Nutrition. 2012;**108**(1):1-8

[61] Stangl GI, Kirchgessner M. Different degrees of moderate iron deficiency modulate lipid metabolism of rats. Lipids. 1998;**33**(9):889-895

[62] Choi JW, Kim SK, Pai SH. Changes in serum lipid concentrations during iron depletion and after iron supplementation. Annals of Clinical and Laboratory Science. 2001;**31**(2):151-156

[63] Özdemir A, Sevinç C, Selamet U, Türkmen F. The relationship between iron deficiency anemia and lipid metabolism in premenopausal women. The American Journal of the Medical Sciences. 2007;**334**(5):331-333

[64] Kamei A, Watanabe Y, Ishijima T, Uehara M, Arai S, Kato H, et al. Dietary iron-deficient anemia induces a variety of metabolic changes and even apoptosis in rat liver: A DNA microarray study. Physiological Genomics. 2010;**42**(2):149-156

[65] Buysschaert M, Paris I, Selvais P, Hermans MP. Clinical aspects of diabetes secondary to idiopathic haemochromatosis in French-speaking Belgium. Diabetes & Metabolism. 1997;**23**(4):308-313

[66] Micha R, Wallace SK, Mozaffarian D. Red and processed meat consumption and risk of incident coronary heart disease, stroke, and diabetes: A systematic review and meta-analysis. Circulation. 2010;**121**(21):2271-2283

[67] Fu S, Li F, Zhou J, Liu Z. The relationship between body iron status, iron intake and gestational diabetes: A systematic review and meta-analysis. Medicine. 2016;**95**(2):e2383

[68] Tiedge M, Lortz S, Drinkgern J, Lenzen S. Relation between antioxidant enzyme gene expression and antioxidative defense status of insulin-producing cells. Diabetes. 1997;**46**(11):1733-1742

[69] Huang J, Jones D, Luo B, Sanderson M, Soto J, Abel ED, et al. Iron overload and diabetes risk: A shift from glucose to fatty acid oxidation and increased hepatic glucose production in a mouse model of hereditary hemochromatosis. Diabetes. 2011;**60**(1):80-87

[70] Swaminathan S, Fonseca VA, Alam MG, Shah SV. The role of iron in diabetes and its complications. Diabetes Care. 2007;**30**(7):1926-1933

[71] Rajpathak S, Ma J, Manson J, Willett WC, Hu FB. Iron intake and the risk of type 2 diabetes in women: A prospective cohort study. Diabetes Care. 2006;**29**(6):1370-1376

[72] Hua NW, Stoohs RA, Facchini FS. Low iron status and enhanced insulin sensitivity in lacto-ovo vegetarians. The British Journal of Nutrition. 2007;**86**(04):515

[73] Ascherio A, Rimm EB, Giovannucci E, Willett WC, Stampfer MJ. Blood donations and risk of coronary heart disease in men. Circulation. 2001;**103**(1):52-57

[74] Valenti L, Fracanzani AL, Dongiovanni P, Rovida S, Rametta R, Fatta E, et al. A randomized trial of iron depletion in patients with nonalcoholic fatty liver disease and hyperferritinemia. World Journal of Gastroenterology. 2014;**20**(11):3002-3010

[75] O'Brien J, Powell LW. Non-alcoholic fatty liver disease: Is iron relevant? Hepatology International. 2012;**6**(1):332-341

[76] Laine F, Ruivard M, Loustaud-Ratti V, Bonnet F, Cales P, Bardou-Jacquet E, et al. Metabolic and hepatic effects of bloodletting in dysmetabolic iron overload syndrome: A randomized controlled study in 274 patients. Hepatology (Baltimore, Md). 2017;**65**(2):465-474

[77] Carmena R, Ascaso JF. Global therapy of diabetic dyslipidemia: Benefits and new therapeutic approaches. Medicina Clinica. 2010;**134**(9):406-411

[78] Taskinen MR. Diabetic dyslipidaemia: From basic research to clinical practice. Diabetologia. 2003;**46**(6):733-749

[79] Haffner SM, Valdez RA, Hazuda HP, Mitchell BD, Morales PA, Stern MP. Prospective analysis of the insulin-resistance syndrome (syndrome X). Diabetes. 1992;**41**(6):715-722

[80] Garcia-Quismondo A. Proteína C reactiva, índice de conicidad y factores de riesgo cardiovascular en pacientes con diabetes tipo 2 [Thesis]. Madrid: Complutense University; 2016

[81] Boizel R, Benhamou PY, Lardy B, Laporte F, Foulon T, Halimi S. Ratio of triglycerides to HDL cholesterol is an indicator of LDL particle size in patients with type 2 diabetes and normal HDL cholesterol levels. Diabetes Care. 2000;**23**(11):1679-1685

[82] Rainwater DL. Lipoprotein correlates of LDL particle size. Atherosclerosis. 2000;**148**(1):151-158

[83] Coppack SW, Evans RD, Fisher RM, Frayn KN, Gibbons GF, Humphreys SM, et al. Adipose tissue metabolism in obesity: Lipase action in vivo before and after a mixed meal. Metabolism: Clinical and Experimental. 1992;**41**(3):264-272

[84] Lee C, Liese A, Wagenknecht L, Lorenzo C, Haffner S, Hanley A. Fish consumption, insulin sensitivity and beta-cell function in the Insulin Resistance Atherosclerosis Study (IRAS). Nutrition, Metabolism and Cardiovascular Diseases. 2013;**23**(9):829-835

[85] Pérez-Granados AM, Vaquero MP, Navarro MP. Sunflower oil versus olive oil and iron metabolism in rats. Influence of a frying process. Journal of the Science of Food and Agriculture. 2001;**81**:115-120

[86] Droke EA, Lukaski HC. Dietary fatty acids and minerals. In: Chow CH, editor. Fatty Acids in Foods and Their Health Implications. 3rd ed. . Boca Raton: CRC Press; 2008. pp. 631-650

[87] Martín de Santa-Olalla L, Sánchez-Muniz FJ, Vaquero MP. N-3 fatty acids in glucose metabolism and insulin sensitivity. Nutrición Hospitalaria. 2009;**24**(2):113-127

[88] Evert AB, Boucher JL, Cypress M, et al. Nutrition therapy recommendations for the management of adults with diabetes. Diabetes Care. 2013;**36**(11):3821-3842

[89] Rametta R, Dongiovanni P, Pelusi S, Francione P et al. Hepcidin resistance in dysmetabolic iron overload. Liver International. 2016;**36**:1540-1548